Synthesis Lectures on Technology and Health

The series publishes state-of-the-art short books on transformative technologies for health, wellness, and independent living. Our scope of publishing in the expanding health tech field includes:

- Technology in support of active and healthy living and aging
- Digital technologies for health- and social-care improvement
- Diagnostic, screening, and tracking tools
- Assistive and rehabilitative technologies

The series includes a subseries of books published in partnership with Canada's AGE-WELL NCE that specifically addresses their 8 AgeTech Challenge Areas. Each lecture introduces the context in which the technology is used—wellness, health, medicine, special needs, or other contexts. Authors present and explain the technology and review promising applications and opportunities as well as limitations and challenges. They include material on their own work while surveying the broader landscape of related research, development, and impact.

LouAnne Boyd

The Sensory Accommodation Framework for Technology

Bridging Sensory Processing to Social Cognition

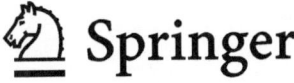 Springer

LouAnne Boyd
Chapman University
Orange, CA, USA

ISSN 2771-7054 ISSN 2771-7070 (electronic)
Synthesis Lectures on Technology and Health
ISBN 978-3-031-48842-9 ISBN 978-3-031-48843-6 (eBook)
https://doi.org/10.1007/978-3-031-48843-6

This Springer imprint is published by the registered company Springer Nature Switzerland AG
The registered company address is: Gewerbestrasse 11, 6330 Cham, Switzerland

Paper in this product is recyclable.

To my sun and my moon, Alex and Natalie.

Acknowledgements

There are so many people I would like to thank for their support in this endeavor. Ten years of my research have culminated in this book. First and foremost, I'd like to thank my advisor Gillian Hayes who has supported me through so many growth experiences, changed my career, and changed my world. Secondly, I would like to thank all my lab mates at Star Lab at UCI where I worked with Gillian and so many talented scholars. All of you have touched my thinking in so many ways and I am so thankful for being able to walk along the path with you for a bit and still being inspired by you all even when far away. More directly, I'd like to thank my academic peers: Franceli Cibrian, Jazette Johnson, Annuska Zolyomi, Kate Ringland, and Mark Baldwin. Over the years we have shared so for their many discussions about this framework at various stages. As this research for the book occurred over 9 years, there are several families and participants that I could thank but they need to remain anonymous; they are etched in gold in my heart. I thank you and along with that all the clinicians that I worked alongside. As I transitioned from a clinician myself into the world of assistive technology, I had the pleasure of working alongside Derek Prate, Eliza DelPizzo-Chang, Sara Jones, Karen Lotich, Hollis pass, Deanna Hughes, Vincent Berardi, MaryBeth Grant-Beuttler, Rahul Sonagra, Kevin Peterson, and RJ De Ramas.

I would also like to thank my dear friends who listen to me talk about this book probably much longer than they care to but, without their careful ears, I would not have been able to process these concepts in the way that I did and for that I'm so grateful. Thank you so much Jennifer LeGault, Julee Nishimi, Barbara Axelsson, Maria Hettinga, Leigh Friedman, and Debbie Kroenberg. I am so very grateful also to Leigh Friedman for her beautiful illustrations of the Social Accommodation Framework for Technology. Her ability to take a vision inside my head and put it on paper in such a beautiful way makes me so very happy.

Lastly, I like to thank the plethora of graduate and undergraduate research assistants that participated in research projects that impacted my thinking about this work: Viseth Sean, Riya Mody, Saumya Gupta, Sagar Bipin Vikmani, Korayma Arriaga, Kim Klein, Kanika Patel, Helen Tomimbang, Andrea Toledo-Conejo, Drew Bozarth, Daniel Dinh, Kevan Parang, Abby Tan, Ayra Tusneem, Alex Muse, Bryce Purnell, Ben Wasserman, Brandon Makin, Kaitlyn Abdo, Alex Hamel, Zach Jagoda, Samantha Gonzalez, Nick Lai, Filip Augustowski, Jack DeBruyn Kai Itoazu, and Cyrus Faamafoe.

Contents

Introduction to Autism for Assistive Technologists

The Birth of Disability

The disabled experience is less common than the norm and less understood (leading to fear of the unknown) thus often becomes stigmatized within each culture (Goffman, 2009). This "uncertainty of what is expected" between able-bodied and disabled bodies (Berger & Wilber, 2013) results in perspectives on the human experience from the able bodies viewing the disabled and the disabled viewing the abled. The disabled view is that these norms that stigmatize are socially constructed by society for the purpose of exclusion (Berger & Wilber, 2013). The able-bodied view, referred to as "the essentialist view", "medical model" (Berger & Wilber, 2013) or "deficit model" (Harry & Klingner, 2007) focuses on deficits from the perceived norm.

From the start of medicine as a field or discipline, this orientation towards disability has been to alleviate the symptoms that lead to human experiences that lie outside the expected norms, often referred to as the "medical model of disability" (Marks, 1997). Underlying this rationale is that the disabled experience must be somehow "less than" the abled body experience; therefore it should be remedied so that one's quality of life is improved (Berger & Wilber, 2013). The medical model of disability has often spilled into other areas, such as education and parenting, in which impairment and "cure" become the focus. Henceforth, dozens of disciplines have emerged along with views that range from the contrary to complementing views of the disabled experience. Disability advocates, allies, and others have critiqued this medical model (e.g., Gillespie-Lynch et al., 2017; Guberman & Haimson, 2023; Mankoff et al., 2010; Williams & Gilbert, 2019, 2020; Woods & Waldock, 2021), the history of which is now a fractured history of assistive technology and one of disciplinary debate.

© The Author(s), under exclusive license to Springer Nature Switzerland AG 2024
L. Boyd, *The Sensory Accommodation Framework for Technology*, Synthesis Lectures on Technology and Health, https://doi.org/10.1007/978-3-031-48843-6_1

History of Autism as a Diagnosis

Autism has been a part of the human experience for as long as there have been records by humans (Silberman, 2015), however the medical diagnosis was not developed in the 1940's (Rosen et al., 2021). Two medical doctors, Kanner and Aspergers, are credited for "discovering" autism (Rosen et al., 2021)]. As a diagnostic category, it has iterated through names such as Autism (American Psychiatric Association, 1987), Pervasive Developmental Disorders, including the introduction of Asperger syndrome (Frances et al., 1995), with inclusion and differentiation of Aspergers syndrome, and Autism Spectrum Disorder (Regier et al., 2013). In the United States, inclusion criteria was first decided across 3 dimensions: social, communication, and behavior. As of this writing, updates to the DSM consist of 2 arms of symptoms that make up the diagnosis: social communication difficulties and restricted, repetitive behaviors (Regier et al., 2013).

Substantial funding has been allocated by the United States government and private agencies alike to determine genetic, epigenetic, prenatal, and environmental factors, to determine autism (Yoon et al., 2020). Autism has been explored by many angles from the once-hypothesized attachment difficulties due to an emotionally deprived environment (e.g., Bethelhem's assertions of "refrigerator moms" as a cause of autism (Mccullough & Ressler, 2018) to genetics (Folstein & Rutter, 1977), to the physical environment (e.g. embryonic and environmental allergens) (Ornoy et al., 2015). Differences in the microbiome in the gut has been found in autistic children (Sivamaruthi et al., 2020). Many disciplines have a focus in relation to related impairments with corresponding discipline-specific interventions. Additionally, pseudo-scientific enterprises have promised cures, *cure du jour* (Goldstein & Ozonoff, 2018). Given the breadth of partial and conflicting information regarding autism, there is a need for a synthesis of all approaches starting with the beginning..

History of Autism's Clinical Interventions

Attributes of an autistic learning style, and impairments of learning that are associated with autism consist of delayed or disorders speech (Cantiani et al., 2016; Kamio et al., 2007; Mundy et al., 1987; Stevenson et al., 2017), (see more in Communication subsection) disorder; diverse or delayed cognitive processes with a focus on deficits in Theory of Mind (inferential thinking) and social cognition (Baron-Cohen, 2001), Executive Functioning (Happé et al., 2006), as well as poorer performance in academic specific achievements such as reading, writing, and math (Bullen et al., 2022). Autism interventions from a therapeutic perspective aim to improve skills or processes that occur within the person. In other words, if autism is believed to occur *inside the body,* then the medical model's goal will focus on ways to improve the ailment within the person. Disciplines have divided up the body and mind into physical parts where each discipline applies their knowledge of the body to produce interventions for autism at their respective level of expertise, with the understanding that crossing these disciplinary boundaries is not sanctioned. In fact, ethics boards exist for each discipline to determine what types of interventions fall within each discipline's purview. This can be confusing for a consumer of medical services to know what lies within each discipline's purview and more importantly why they do not seem to have very little overlap, see Fig. 1.1.

For example, **psychiatry**, psychology, and cognitive science are all concerned with the mind, the brain, and neurons. These concepts refer to the same body part but have widely different approaches. In the division of interventions, Psychiatry manages psycho-tropic medication management (believing autism is a chemical imbalance in the brain). Currently there is no medication to treat autism, yet several medications, and at times, a cocktail of medications are prescribed to address related symptoms such as depression, anxiety,

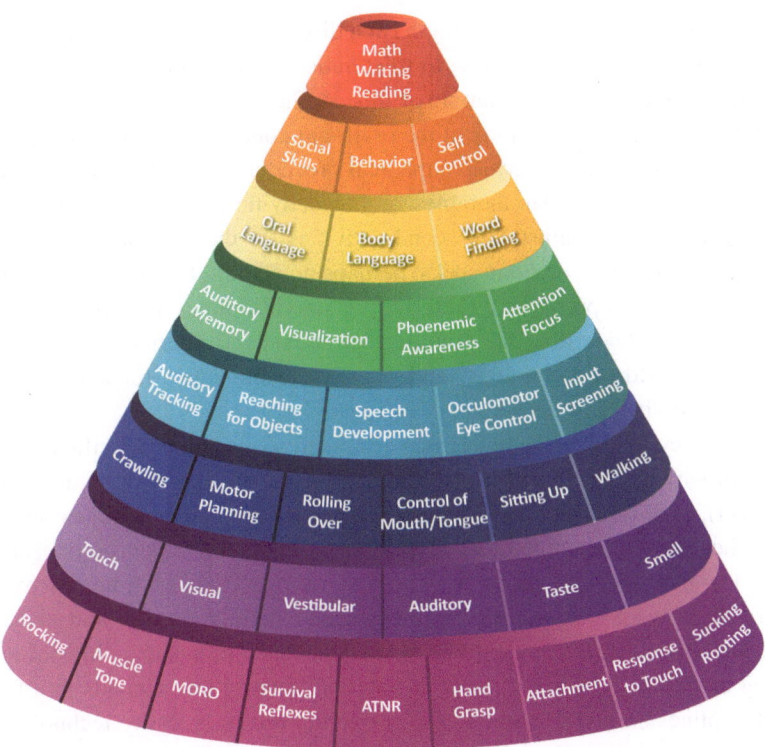

Fig. 1.1 Learning cone inspired by the learning skills pyramid. For source and interactive example from clinical perspective see link: https://www.hol-solutions.com/learning-challenges/learning-skills-pyramid/

explosive behaviors, seizures, and ADHD (Spencer et al., 2013). Psychologists also provide psychotherapy but usually from a cognitive or behavioral perspective in relation to autism (implying that autism can be unlearned or trained out of existence).

Special education and related services such as, Behavior Analysis, Speech Language Pathology, Occupational Therapy, Physical Therapy take the deficit model approach from the perspective of their disipline's focus by supplying teaching and training of "developmental skills" that are the core of the education program. These are skills that are acquired during the early course of a child's development and expected to occur naturally over specified periods of time. These interventions take the form of special education in classrooms, specialized learning, and parent training, speech and communication therapy, training in daily living skills (such as fine motor skills, dressing, eating), sensory integration therapy, large motor skills (such as walking), respectively. Even more disciplines and non-medical approaches have taken an interest in autism, however the challenge is who they can be integrated with.

Disciplines, as well as the people within each discipline, may differ in their belief about what causes autism and therefore how to treat autism, thus resulting in interventions that may contradict one another. An example of this conflict is the approach to treating autism by the bio-medical doctors who look at the brain-gut connection as the etiology of autism and ascribe to a strict series of invasive medical procedures that leave little room, energy, time, money, support for other therapies or life activities. This approach is a lifestyle that can be isolating for mainstream social activities for the child and family members. However, if a cure is what someone seeks, perhaps no amount of intervention is too much. With this vast array of approaches, these segregated disciplines seeped into the world of assistive technology. Over time the "industry of autism" (Broderick, & Roscigno, 2021) has entered the world of technology, and assistive technologies for autism have grown substantially in the last few decades.

Each discipline attributes characteristics of autism to discipline-specific causes such as atypical brain wiring, interfering gut toxins, lack of knowledge, lack of motivation (e.g., reinforcement), lack of sensory integration. Each discipline also operates on a different temporal schedule for example, the behavioral and learning sciences expect a certain amount of learning and or mastery to occur in short periods of time where as a may take several days weeks or months to change one's cellular health, and and then even longer for the GroundTruth change to be observable, such as a change in communication. As learning can occur over short temporal intervals from a few seconds to a few weeks, learning disciplines are viable candidates for making analog assistive technologies which are generally focused on seeing changes in behavior in a relatively short period of time— that aligns with the ethos of technology—fast results.

Introduction of Human–Computer Interaction (HCI) to Autism

HCI as a field, however does not ascribe to a specific epistemology of Autism, rather it is often the individual HCI researchers who defer to their stakeholders-which varies from project to project–discipline to discipline-therapeutic to assistive-thus making it confusing to generate a canon of literature that has the same goal. Autism has been the focus for technologists to diagnose, treat biomedical deficiencies, survey deficits, rehabilitate, train, teach, keep separate to keep safe, to leverage strengths, provide a critical perspective, and to celebrate diversity. Since the onset of interactive technologies for autism, the number and robustness has grown tremendously (Kientz et al., 2013). Across a variety of platforms, early interactive technologies targeted communication, social-emotional, academic, life skills, vocational, sensory motor, and restricted and repetitive behavior (Kientz et al., 2013). Still today, the majority of autism technologies come from the perspective of the medical model, however a social model of autism has led to some work from an end user's perspective via a Disability Studies perspective.

The Birth of the Neurodiversity Movement (And Its Impact on HCI)

The complexity of an autism label requires analysis of the "dynamics between diagnosis, identity, power, and inclusion" (Zolyomi & Tennis, 2017). Autistics may embrace an identity of autism and still take up medical model services to address symptoms they wish to remediate, thus brushing up against a range of opposing epistemes, as described in Part 1 (Fig. 1.2).

In Favor of Autistic Goals and Needs

From the work of autistic disability studies scholars, several symptoms of autism are of interest in the area of intervention. According to (Williams & Gilbert, 2020), these include supporting issues such as emotional and sensory regulation, communication, motor coordination, executive functioning and sensory processing. A few studies have addressed these areas. For example, the design of wearable applications has been explored to support self-control of behavior of children with ADHD, however this application has not deployed yet (Cibrian et al., 2020). Other projects have explored the use of multisensory interactive displays as a therapeutic to support the motor development and sensory processing integration of autistic children found that natural user interfaces in tandem with multi-sensory stimuli are easy to use and useful for children with severe autism (Ringland et al., 2014).

These approaches consider the whole human and beyond at societal level. Disability Studies is a formal "discipline" that sheds light on the macro level of human experience,

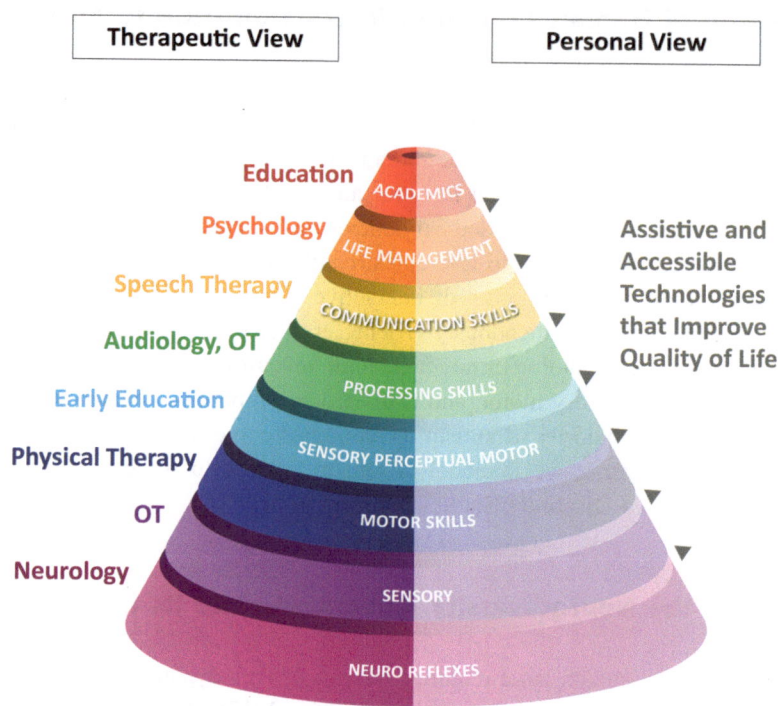

Fig. 1.2 Learning cone from two perspectives (Therapeutic vs. Personal)

rather than specific impairments of the individual. Alternative theory of autism that aims to understand the autistic expression as a whole from the perspective of those with autism is Monotropism. Monotropism is a theory of autism by autistics to explain the autism experience as a whole person with singular interests (Murray et al., 2005) that involves the strong tendency "to localize and concentrate to the exclusion of other input; an atypicality from which many other differences can be seen to follow. Understanding this concept fully requires a view of the mind as a system of interests which inform cognitive, perceptual, and emotional processes" (Murray, 2018).

In Fig. 1.3, I have illustrated several examples of technology pointed at the user's behavior change and pointed at changes in the world of the user. Starting with the top of the cone at the academics ring, to the left, we have the disciplines approach to managing reading issues. A clinician or educator might want to change the pronunciation of words in a particular student. They might provide feedback on a word by word basis, or develop technology that will give feedback about pronunciation. This is pointed at the user's feedback as for the user to take in and make changes. On the other side, there's an arrow pointing out from academics on how to change the world for the user. An example of a technology here would be automating the color of a background to make reading more visible therefore easier for the user. The burden of change is on the technology to change

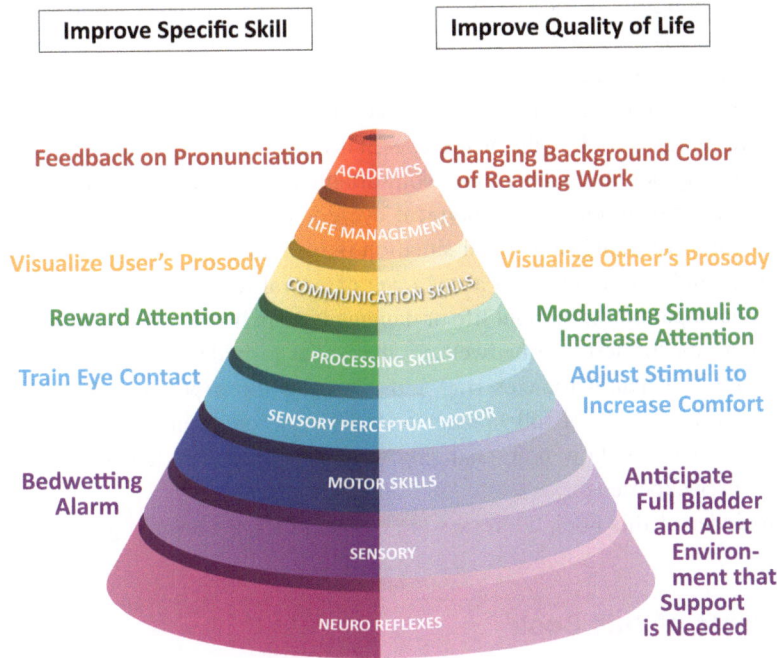

Fig. 1.3 Example of goals of technology from two perspectives

the environment and make things easier. Ultimately, the goal is the same with the users reading improving, and with the outward pointing version, the user is also likely to be more comfortable.

The second example is on the communication ring. On the left, the behavior to change is the user's prosody. The technology that visualizes the users prosody thus provides feedback to the user on how well they performed. On the right side where the arrow is leaving the communication ring and facing out into the world. That communication goal would be to visualize others prosody, therefore giving the user a view of prosody in use in the world without burdening them to attend to technology and also the pressure to change a deeply rooted behavior.

The third example is on the processing skills ring. To the left eye technology might be aimed at rewarding attention to a task via a watch or another wearable or something tracking eye gaze. On the right, the scale that comes out from the processing scale ring into the world would be augmenting the stimuli to be more attention worthy in other words, making it more easily consumed for attention, such as filtering visual aspects.

The fourth example is at the sensory perception level. On the left, the arrow is pointing in towards sensory perception and states one may be training eye contact using a technology like a desktop computer, where the camera is monitoring eye contact, and giving life feedback or recorded feedback for later review. Again, this feedback is about the users' performance leaving the burden of change up to the user to manage while also attending to whatever content they're intended to be looking at. On the right, the arrow leaving sensory perception out into the world, shows the technology might modulate the viewing of triggering stimuli. In autism, eye contact has been described as painful, therefore rather than training to look right at the eyes, an outwarding pointing technology could change the environment to make it more comfortable to view people without targeting the eyes. The result may resemble neurotypical eye contact behavior but more importantly, the user's comfort of being in a social situation is increased.

The last example in the figure is at the level of neural reflexes. These develop early in life, but can be impaired throughout life or damage later in life. Example for a clinical goal and technology on the left is a bedwetting alarm that provides feedback after urination. The air leaving the neural reflexes ring and changing the experience of the world is a technology that anticipates a full bladder and alerts the environment for support. These examples are meant to show how changing the orientation of a technology can greatly improve the user experience.

The remainder of this book addresses the details of these research gaps.

The Contents of this Book

This book is designed to provide a detailed overview of several aspects of technology for autism. Each Chapter contains figures to illustrate different parts of the Sensory Accommodation Framework. This first Chapter discusses a variety of skills that make up human development, see Fig. 1.4a. The Chapter also provides a history of autism as a diagnosis as well as the birth of the neurodiversity movement. Details about education and clinician focus regarding developmental domains are detailed in relation to existing technologies to support these aims, see Fig. 1.4b. This Chapter also discusses an Autistic User-First perspective of assistive technologies and potential goals. The clinical and a personal view are contrasted and imp;ictoosn for bridging three perspectives is provided, see Fig. 1.4c.

In Chap. 2, more details are provided about the individual types of therapy and how they interact with autism. Examples of technologies that are driven by these therapy goals are also provided. Recommendations for user experience goals are discussed as well, see Fig. 1.4d.

Chapter 3 details the systems involved in sensory processing and how they relate to autism specifically. Again, examples of technologies that have addressed these areas are provided and an illustration of the sensory of first approach is provided in Fig. 1.4e. Applications for designers are also provided.

In Chap. 4, designing sensory environments and sensory interactions and virtual reality is discussed through a virtual reality project. Design details are discussed for five virtual realities that each focus on a certain sensory persona based on Dunn's sensory profiles. These are based on individuals' neurological thresholds and self-regulation behaviors.

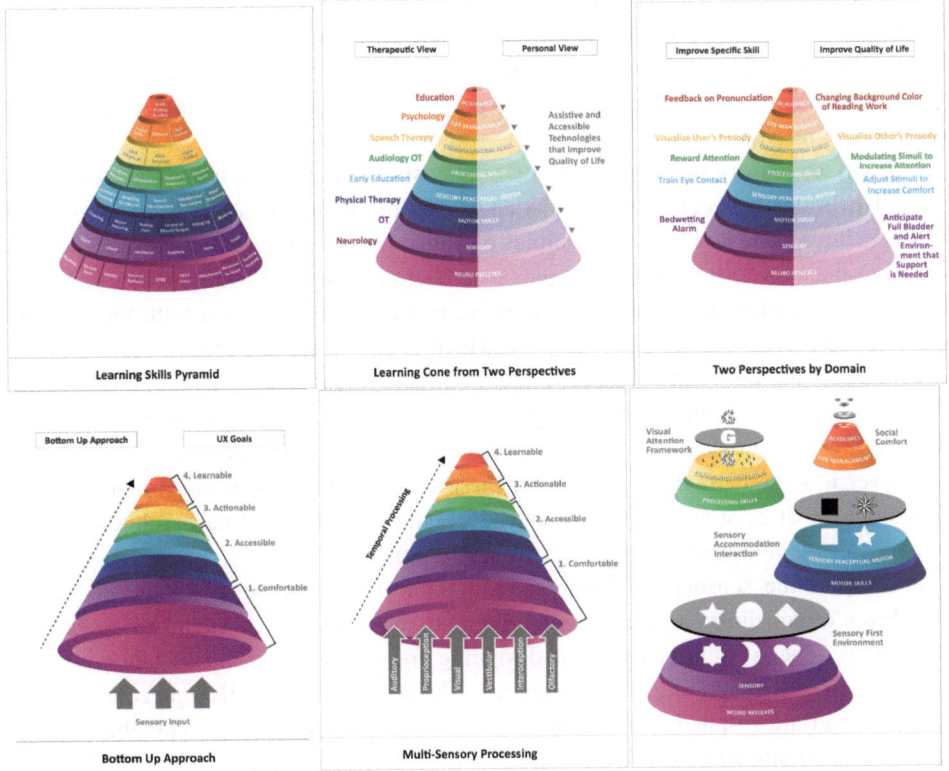

Fig. 1.4 Summary of models from each chapter

Two layers of the sensory accommodation framework are discussed in this Chapter. The first is closer to the bottom of the learning cone and that is the sensory environments model, see Fig. 1.4f. Additionally the next layer up in the learning cone involves motor and sensory processing and this is discussed in terms of sensory interactions. Strategies for managing these in assistive technologies are discussed as well, see Fig. 1.4g. Input from previous Chapters is applied to these Chapters as the suggestions move up through the processing pathways.

In Chap. 5, visual attention and how it is related and different in autism as well as some other neurodivergent conditions such as ADHD and dyslexia is examined. The hierarchy of information that is often not discussed in technology is discussed in depth in this Chapter. Global and local information, how it relates to eye gaze and impacts visual attention or discussed as well as a case example through a project called the global filter. The next layer of the sensory accommodation framework is pictured which is a way to filter out in highlighting Global Information or provide indication of what the structure is of information and what to attend to in terms of understanding the gist of a natural scene.

See Fig. 1.4h. Chapter 5 also discusses how to apply the global filter to an AAC device for people with Autism who may not only benefit from the highlighted Global Information in terms of improving receptive communication comprehension, and the device concept also provides expressive communication options based on what has been indicated as semantically relevant.

In Chap. 6, sensory perception and its relationship to nonverbal communication is the focus. The bridge between sensory input and social behavior is discussed. Dynamic information is introduced and several examples of nonverbal communication and Technologies related to them are mentioned. Examples from technologies that demonstrate the mechanisms for supporting memorable communication are provided. Along with the top layer of the sensory accommodation framework which is called social comfort, see Fig. 1.4i.

In Chap. 7 the information processing system is complicated by temporal processing. More discussion of multisensory integration is provided and examples of ADHD and dyslexia are also provided in terms of how sensory information becomes more complicated over time and strategies to support these learning differences are provided. Again technologies that exist are mentioned as well as strategies to build new technologies, see Fig. 1.4j for the temporal multisensory processing model.

In Chap. 8 the sensory accommodation framework is summarized in terms of how each layer offers different user experience goals and specific mechanisms to promote those goals. The recommendation of designing from the bottom up to make sure that each level is well supported by the previous level is reiterated. Design considerations for each level are restated and a summary or overview of the design guidelines for the Sensory Accommodation Framework are provided. See Fig. 1.4k.

References

American Psychiatric Association. (1987). *Diagnostic and statistical manual of... Book by American osychiatric association* (3rd revised ed.).

Baron-Cohen, S. (2001). "Reading the mind in the eyes" test revised version: A study with normal adults, and adults with asperger syndrome or high-functioning autism. *Journal of Child Psychology and Psychiatry, 42*(2), 241–251.

Berger, R. J. & Wilber, L. (2013). *Introducing disability studies.* Lynne Rienner Publishers.

Broderick, A. A., & Roscigno, R. (2021). Autism, Inc.: The autism industrial complex. *Journal of Disability Studies in Education.* https://brill.com/view/journals/jdse/2/1/article-p77_77.xml

Bullen, J. C., Zajic, M. C., McIntyre, N., Solari, E., & Mundy, P. (2022). Patterns of math and reading achievement in children and adolescents with autism spectrum disorder. *Research in Autism Spectrum Disorders, 92*, 101933. https://doi.org/10.1016/j.rasd.2022.101933

Cantiani, C., Choudhury, N. A., Yu, Y. H., Shafer, V. L., Schwartz, R. G., & Benasich, A. A. (2016). From sensory perception to lexical-semantic processing: An ERP study in non-verbal children with autism. *PLoS ONE, 11*(8), e0161637. https://doi.org/10.1371/journal.pone.0161637

Cibrian, F. L., Lakes, K. D., Tavakoulnia, A., Guzman, K., Schuck, S., & Hayes, G. R. (2020). Supporting self-regulation of children with ADHD using wearables: Tensions and design challenges. In *Proceedings of the 2020 CHI conference on human factors in computing systems* (pp. 1–13).

Folstein, S., & Rutter, M. (1977). Infantile autism: A genetic study of 21 twin Pairs. *Journal of Child Psychology and Psychiatry, 18*(4), 297–321. https://doi.org/10.1111/j.1469-7610.1977.tb00443.x

Frances, A., First, M. B., & Pincus, H. A. (1995). *DSM-IV guidebook* (pp. x, 501). American Psychiatric Association.

Gillespie-Lynch, K., Kapp, S. K., Brooks, P. J., Pickens, J., & Schwartzman, B. (2017). Whose expertise is it? Evidence for autistic adults as critical autism experts. *Frontiers in Psychology, 8*. https://www.frontiersin.org/articles/10.3389/fpsyg.2017.00438

Goffman, E. (2009). *Stigma: Notes on the management of spoiled identity.* Simon and Schuster.

Goldstein, S., & Ozonoff, S. (2018). *Assessment of autism spectrum disorder* (2nd ed.). Guilford Publications.

Guberman, J., & Haimson, O. (2023). Not robots; Cyborgs—Furthering anti-ableist research in human-computer interaction. *First Monday.* https://doi.org/10.5210/fm.v28i1.12910

Happé, F., Booth, R., Charlton, R., & Hughes, C. (2006). Executive function deficits in autism spectrum disorders and attention-deficit/hyperactivity disorder: Examining profiles across domains and ages. *Brain and Cognition, 61*(1), 25–39. https://doi.org/10.1016/j.bandc.2006.03.004

Harry, B., & Klingner, J. (2007). Discarding the deficit model. *Educational Leadership, 64*(5), 16.

Kamio, Y., Robins, D., Kelley, E., Swainson, B., & Fein, D. (2007). Atypical lexical/semantic processing in high-functioning autism spectrum disorders without early language delay. *Journal of Autism and Developmental Disorders, 37*(6), 1116–1122. https://doi.org/10.1007/s10803-006-0254-3

Kientz, J. A., Goodwin, M. S., Hayes, G. R., & Abowd, G. D. (2013). Interactive technologies for autism. *Synthesis Lectures on Assistive, Rehabilitative, and Health-Preserving Technologies, 2*(2), 1–177. https://doi.org/10.2200/S00533ED1V01Y201309ARH004

Mankoff, J., Hayes, G. R., & Kasnitz, D. (2010). Disability studies as a source of critical inquiry for the field of assistive technology. In *Proceedings of the 12th international ACM SIGACCESS conference on computers and accessibility* (pp. 3–10). http://dl.acm.org/citation.cfm?id=1878807

Marks, D. (1997). Models of disability. *Disability and Rehabilitation, 19*(3), 85–91. https://doi.org/10.3109/09638289709166831

Mccullough, K., & Ressler, K. (2018). *Posttraumatic stress disorder: From neurobiology to cycles of violence: integrating research, practice, and policy* (pp. 19–54). https://doi.org/10.1007/978-3-030-00503-0_3

Mundy, P., Sigman, M., Ungerer, J., & Sherman, T. (1987). Nonverbal communication and play correlates of language development in autistic children. *Journal of Autism and Developmental Disorders, 17*(3), 349–364. https://doi.org/10.1007/BF01487065

Murray, D. (2018). Monotropism—An interest based account of autism. In *Encyclopedia of autism spectrum disorders.*

Murray, D., Lesser, M., & Lawson, W. (2005). Attention, monotropism and the diagnostic criteria for autism. *Autism, 9*(2), 139–156. https://doi.org/10.1177/1362361305051398

Ornoy, A., Weinstein-Fudim, L., & Ergaz, Z. (2015). Prenatal factors associated with autism spectrum disorder (ASD). *Reproductive Toxicology, 56*, 155–169. https://doi.org/10.1016/j.reprotox.2015.05.007

Regier, D. A., Kuhl, E. A., & Kupfer, D. J. (2013). The DSM-5: Classification and criteria changes. *World Psychiatry, 12*(2), 92–98. https://doi.org/10.1002/wps.20050

Ringland, K. E., Zalapa, R., Neal, M., Escobedo, L., Tentori, M., & Hayes, G. R. (2014). *SensoryPaint: A multimodal sensory intervention for children with neurodevelopmental disorders* (pp. 873–884). https://doi.org/10.1145/2632048.2632065

Rosen, N. E., Lord, C., & Volkmar, F. R. (2021). The Diagnosis of autism: From Kanner to DSM-III to DSM-5 and beyond. *Journal of Autism and Developmental Disorders, 51*(12), 4253–4270. https://doi.org/10.1007/s10803-021-04904-1

Silberman, S. (2015). *Neurotribes: The legacy of autism and the future of neurodiversity.* Penguin.

Sivamaruthi, B. S., Suganthy, N., Kesika, P., & Chaiyasut, C. (2020). The role of microbiome, dietary supplements, and probiotics in autism spectrum disorder. *International Journal of Environmental Research and Public Health, 17*(8), Article 8. https://doi.org/10.3390/ijerph17082647

Spencer, D., Marshall, J., Post, B., Kulakodlu, M., Newschaffer, C., Dennen, T., Azocar, F., & Jain, A. (2013). Psychotropic medication use and polypharmacy in children with autism spectrum disorders. *Pediatrics, 132*(5), 833–840. https://doi.org/10.1542/peds.2012-3774

Stevenson, R. A., Baum, S. H., Segers, M., Ferber, S., Barense, M. D., & Wallace, M. T. (2017). Multisensory speech perception in autism spectrum disorder: From phoneme to whole-word perception. *Autism Research, 10*(7), 1280–1290. https://doi.org/10.1002/aur.1776

Williams, R. M., & Gilbert, J. E. (2019). Cyborg perspectives on computing research reform. In *Extended abstracts of the 2019 CHI conference on human factors in computing systems* (pp. 1–11). https://doi.org/10.1145/3290607.3310421

Williams, R. M., & Gilbert, J. E. (2020). Perseverations of the academy: A survey of wearable technologies applied to autism intervention. *International Journal of Human-Computer Studies, 143*, 102485. https://doi.org/10.1016/j.ijhcs.2020.102485

Woods, R., & Waldock, K. E. (2021). Critical autism studies. In F. R. Volkmar (Ed.), *Encyclopedia of autism spectrum disorders* (pp. 1240–1248). Springer International Publishing. https://doi.org/10.1007/978-3-319-91280-6_102297

Yoon, S. H., Choi, J., Lee, W. J., & Do, J. T. (2020). Genetic and epigenetic etiology underlying autism spectrum disorder. *Journal of Clinical Medicine, 9*(4), Article 4. https://doi.org/10.3390/jcm9040966

Zolyomi, A., & Tennis, J. T. (2017). The autism prism: A domain analysis paper examining neurodiversity. *NASKO*, 139–172. https://doi.org/10.7152/nasko.v6i1.15237

Technologies Across the Disciplines for Autistic Users

2

Introduction

Autism is a lived experience that is complex and offers a rich opportunity for design opportunities across almost every aspect of life—even the positive aspects. There are two main groups of technologies that get built for autism the first being therapeutic or educational the second grouping assistive or accessible. Several disciplines contribute as domain experts in assistive technologies for autism. For example in (Kientz et al., 2013), technology has been developed to address features of autism, such as developing innovative diagnosis tools, developing tools to support education, recreation, leisure, and social communication. Many tools target personal independence as an optimal outcome. To spite the breath of attention given to autism, there has not been a synthesized approach to pull the various disciplines and communities together.

Although the disciplines of medicine, psychology, and psychiatry branch off from with the initial movement to secure safety for the masses in a time when the mechanism of spreading disease was not well understood. Back then, separating people with symptoms that were different/unknown was group with those symptoms that were possibly contagious. Diseased and disabled people were siloed from society, thus removing explanation of the lived experience from the disabled perspective. Over time, disciples for specific conditions were formed and each discipline drew boundaries around certain impairments described in an autism diagnosis. Treatments to address these varied impairments were then based on the focus of discipline-specific domains, although some skills-such as attention- are taken up by a variety of disciplines. How each field engages with autism is through the lens of their discipline. See Fig. 2.1.

L. Boyd, *The Sensory Accommodation Framework for Technology*, Synthesis Lectures on Technology and Health, https://doi.org/10.1007/978-3-031-48843-6_2

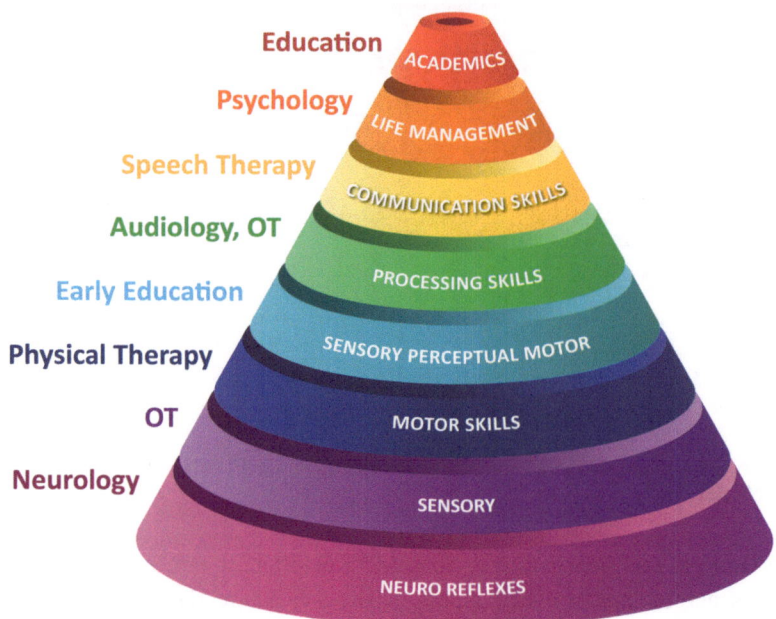

Fig. 2.1 Learning cone with disciplines

Disciplines and Autism Diagnosis

Understanding disease, disorders, and disability gave rise to regulated approaches known as "disciplines" each with their own focus on how to rehabilitate conditions that fall outside the norm. With the crisis of world wars, classification systems for census purposes as well as to evaluate the suitability of men for war (*DSM History*, n.d.). In 1977, the Diagnostics and Statistical Manual (DSM) was developed to house criteria for determining what was considered a mental disorder(*DSM History*, n.d.). The discipline of Education followed suit and created special education programs for those who were and were not previously deemed educatable (Martin et al., 1996). With disabled people living among the mainstream, classifications became prescriptive for school and health programs. A diagnosis of autism meant something specific to a variety of autism stakeholders—be it insight into their loved one's behavior or access to resources. Autism became an eligibility category for special education in 1990 (Pennington et al., 2014). Median rates of autism globally have been estimated between 2012 and 2022 as 100 per 10,000 (Zeidan et al., 2022).

Special Education

The field of special education in the United States serves children ages 0–21 years with a variety of disabilities. From the top of the learning skills pyramid, academics or education as a field views learning as an age-related developmental process. When people fall outside to meet age-related standards they are deemed advanced or delayed. The word choice of "delayed" has a connotation of the potential to catch up to the average range which is the implied promise of Special Education—to remediate developmental gaps. The explanation of autism is that autism is amenable to learning normative behavior. Thus the goals of education specialists in relation to autism is to determine a free and appropriate placement (and support the diverse learning needs so that each student may reach toward their academic potential (Apling & Jones, 2001). Individualized interventions for autism, general special education techniques, and strength-based approaches have been devised to meet these aims (Abosi & Koay, 2008).

Common educational goals for autistic children center around the core curriculum of reading, writing and math. Autistic participants tend to write less than neurotypical participants with errors particularly in spelling and organization, resulting in less efficient written communication (Accardo et al., 2020). A parallel difficulty appears to occur in reading as well. Many technological interventions have been dedicated to dyslexia that address the form of language in terms of fonts and visual processing (more on that in later Chapters) (Boros et al., 2016; Del Valle Rubido et al., 2018; Franceschini et al., 2017; Goldstein-Marcusohn et al., 2020; Rello & Baeza-Yates, 2016; Rello & Bigham, 2017; Stein, 2014; Tsermentseli et al., 2008; Vidyasagar, 2004).This difficulty is carried over into arithmetic as well where researchers have found that autistic children may struggle with problem solving even though they may calculate correctly (Chiang & Lin, 2007). Splintering of reading, writing, and math skills may occur as well where students may perform the same as age-matched peers for one scale but be significantly below for another (Bullen et al., 2022).

Applied Behavior Analysis

Applied Behavior Analysis (ABA) is a branch of psychology that incorporates learning science principles. One of the primary goals of ABA is engineering the environment to promote learning via techniques such as reinforcement, error correction and prompting (Abdo & Al Osman, 2019; Knight et al., 2013). The systematic approach of behavior analysis at first glance appears to be well suited to be readily adaptable to automation. ABA intervention is financially expensive, therefore "extending resources using technology to support learning provides additional motivation" (Abdo & Al Osman, 2019).

Communication

The population of people who have a diagnosis of Autism has a significant portion of minimally verbal people. These people may receive speech services to address speaking or otherwise using a system to communicate sounds, words, and sentences. Some technologies that aim to support this effort are the Spoken Impact project (Hailpern et al., 2009) and VocSyl (Hailpern et al., 2010) to stimulate any vocalization via visualization. However, the communication difficulties that seem to be unique to autism are the ability to learn individual words and spelling and rules of language, yet have difficulty putting it all together to comprehend the meaning–be that at the sentence level or a grander scale (Jolliffe & Baron-Cohen, 1999). This claim is well supported by researchers, who have explored a pattern of autistic children with impaired comprehension of sentences but not of single words (Prior & Hall, 1979).

There is also the dual nature of language, where it is more than words that are employed to convey meaning (e.g., nonverbal communication). Some projects that aim to visualize the unspoken aspects of communication include ProCom which was a functional prototype of a wearable aimed to communicate the users proximity to others by color coding social norms (Boyd et al., 2017), sayWAT, a visual prompt on google glass when interlocutors used a loud or flat tone of voice (Boyd et al., 2016), and vrSocial which was a virtual environment with proximity rings on the ground, a voice-o-meter to visualize how much each person spoke (Boyd et al., 2018). An inclusive design, MOSOCO, involved a mobile phone used to prompt mixed ability students to engage in eye contact, topics of interests, and finding conversation partners (Escobedo et al., 2012).

Psychology

Social cognition involves the integration and pruning of perceptual information; this leads to the formation of an abstract representation (gist). This process takes place within and across different sensory perceptual modalities. Social cognition has been well characterized at the behavioral level, (Henry et al., 2016) and has been measured using tools designed for atypical populations. Four domains of social cognition have been found to be poorer in the autistic population (Henry et al., 2016). Methods to measure these domains involve techniques beyond direct observation and self-report, which can be limited in terms of test–retest and interrater reliability, as well as sensitivity.

Emotion Recognition and Regulation

Emotion recognition is a topic that addresses a space similar to self-regulation and self-monitoring. Historically psychologists have supported emotion recognition and emotion management which also has a strong tie to psychiatric treatment through medication management.

An early system Emotion Bubbles is a system made up of a minicomputer and a camera to detect emotions in real time, (Madsen et al., 2008). The system employed facial analysis software and visualized output to assist autistic youth with understanding and eliciting emotions in conversational peers. Since the uptake of wearable devices, technical solutions to augmenting the process of recognizing emotions include a project called SuperGlass (Washington et al., 2017). Superglass targeted the recognition of the emotions of others via an overlay of an emoji of the people within the wearer's view as well as promoted elicit positive emotions in others via a game of trying to make somebody smile and using the overlaid emotions to see if the wearer was successful. Emotions were detected by an emotion recognition algorithm based on normative facial expressions. Similarly, emotional regulation of one's own behaviors (target skill oriented toward the user's awareness of their emotions) has been explored through EMOglass (Yan et al., 2022). Lastly, mental Health constructs such as anxiety as a target for self-regulation have been parlayed into technologies to prompt users to refer to their logged data for a deeper understanding of the context of triggers. For example, Clasp (Simm et al., 2014) found "Some of the adults with ASD said that they found it difficult to remember when and where they are anxious. If this information was logged using a digital anxiety device linked to their smartphone, then an anxiety history could be seen, showing dates and times they used the device and what triggers were reached". These systems overlap significantly in their aim to support regulation of self as well and awareness of one's surroundings.

Social Skills

Social skills include a broad set of skills that support communication (verbal, and non-verbal), collaboration, understanding others' emotions and managing one's own, and the normative demonstration of affective empathy. Many of these domains have been addressed by technology projects. For example, collaboration between neurodivergent and neurotypical children has been explored. In SIDES, a tabletop display was leveraged to support 4 autistic players with collaborative play (Piper et al., 2006). With an iPad game called Zody's Clock Catastrophe (Boyd et al., 2015), where a sequence of collaborative behaviors were associated with specific game mechanics for school-aged children. Going beyond skill-building for the individual or small group of autistic students includes considering the inclusion of these technologies in mainstream society involves working in mixed ability groups or neurodiverse groups. One work that probes autistic college students about their collaboration in neurodiverse groups found several strategies to support via dozen strategies to support neurodiverse student teams (Zolyomi et al., 2018). Collaborative work extends across the lifespan to include gainful employment. Employment has been explored through a project that promoted Strength-based video modeling for job interviews (Ulgado et al., 2013).

Occupation Therapy

Occupational Therapy is a form of rehabilitation that works with people with developmental delays, physical and cognitive disabilities. They use therapeutic activities to help an individual develop or restore important living skills. For a child, this may include teaching with a child to develop the fine and visual motor/perceptual skills needed to complete self-care tasks, scissor skills, and handwriting to name a few. Sensory processing and sensory integration disorders impact motor planning and sequencing to engage in the management of their daily life in a self-determined manner. Occupational therapy addresses fine motor movements from a developmental perspective, grasp development, pre-writing and writing skills, and bilateral hand coordination skills needed to button a shirt or use scissors for example. Occupational Therapy views autism as delayed or disordered fine motor, motor planning, and sensory integration as well self-advocacy. Therefore, occupational therapy related technologies support a broad range of activities across a lifetime. The routine of brushing teeth can be challenging from a parent's perspective as sensory sensitivities as well as organization and motivation needs may not align with the child's needs. A project that provides visual scaffolding to support the routing of toothbrushes addresses one aspect of daily living (Hayes & Hosaflook, 2013). Other technologies for autism in the occupational therapy discipline focus on sensory processing differences. Sensory processing and sensory integration (processing multiples sensory streams) are foundation features of living. Our sensory system provides feedback about our relationship with self and the environment to support maintaining homeostasis. Technical systems that aim to support sensory processing and sensory integration often customize access to multiple sensory modules. The dominant sensory modules are touch and movement as these sensations were the first to develop in the womb. Additionally visual and auditory modalities take up a large portion of processing in the brain's processing. Managing these inputs at these sensory levels is automatic therefore technologies that aim to support sensory integration do so by allowing for user control and exploration of over multiple modalities. The integration of these modalities is believed to assist with self-regulation and then further down the processing chain, self-monitoring. Technologies that address self-regulation through sensory exploration include MEDIATE, a multisensory environment with large projection screens and audio, audio changes based on body movements (Parés et al., n.d.); Sensory-Paint (Ringland et al., 2014); vrSensory (Boyd, 2019) and BendableSound (Cibrian et al., 2017).

Specifically, regarding sensory overwhelm, CognalityVR is a functional web-based, mobile VR as an accessible option for mediating sensory overload (Boyd et al., 2022), harnessing the power of the internet to reach users beyond the lab. That work deployed a web-based application to use on a smartphone worn in a cardboard headset. "Autistic individuals have an abundance of sensory needs." More often than not, children with autism get overwhelmed or underwhelmed with sensory stimuli, which makes it difficult for them to learn and communicate. It is fundamental that we first address their sensory needs so that, in turn, it is easier for them to process and socialize. Research using virtual reality to address the sensory needs of neurodiverse children showed that even the smallest of details, like the height of a toilet in a virtual environment, can make a huge difference in the experience of the child (Ramachandiran et al., 2015).

Physical Therapy and Orientation and Mobility/Transportation (Mobility Specialists)

Physical therapy is a form of developmental therapy that addresses skill deficits in gross (large) motor movements such as arms and legs; they address gait patterns, proprioception and movement patterns for safety, and core strength in relation to developing norms. As movement is crucial for a sense of independence, addressing movement difficulties through physical therapy presents a set of challenges that can be exacerbated when working with children, especially when physical, sensory, and intellectual disabilities play a role in the complexity for therapy.

Regarding sensory processing, the adoption of atypical movement patterns is increased due to seeking or avoiding behaviors. These atypical patterns may result in strategies that decrease the demands that would be typically placed on the involved muscles. Continuation of atypical movement patterns would then lead to a delay in gross motor skills and ultimately lead to increased safety risks due to weakness in primary muscle groups that are essential for controlling the body when jumping or running. Further along the processing continuum, intellectual abilities may be impacted. For example, difficulties educating the patient and establishing pathways to progressing gross motor skills that would typically develop through play may not be achieved due to the above challenges.

Technologies have been incorporated to enhance motivation for the repetitive skill practice required of physical rehabilitation. One technology project that aimed to provide user feedback to children who toe walk did so through haptic and visual feedback on mobile phones. Smartstepper, (Pollind et al., 2019). Although the participant in this study did not identify as autistic, toe walking is a common trait in autistic children and adults. In the Smartstepper project, the same researcher surveyed the children to understand the impact of toe walking on the quality of their life. They found results ranging from pain to stigma. Future gym visualizes expected proximity between children in a physical education activity to support motor planning and socialization in a group of 20 autistic teens (Takahashi et al., 2018). The Feel and Touch project assessed gestures via haptics for classifying autistic children from remote locations (Monarca et al., 2021, 2023). An interactive sonification system was added to the Go with the Flow system aimed to support movement therapy for autistic children (Cibrian et al., 2021).

Across the lifespan, mobility is extended to getting around a city and some researchers have explored the planning and sensory needs if autistic users as they navigate their surroundings. Wayfinding is a project that augmented details about a location for the purpose of urban navigation (Rapp et al., 2018).

Neurology

Neurologists and psychiatrists, do autism as a differently functioning brain. Their interventions focused, primarily on pharmacology to address brain and behavior. Some concerns of the brain are the potential for epilepsy, and some medications are aimed at reducing the likelihood of epilepsy. Other medications are used to manage behaviors and others are attempting to fix the core neurological deficits, aimed to improve communication and other deficits (Chez et al., 2004).

Therapeutic technologies do not meet all the wants and needs of those with autism or other neurodivergent conditions. Considering the user-centric viewpoint and User Experience Goals for Assistive and Accessible technologies for Autism and other neurodivergencies can help fill the gap, see Fig. 2.2.

Implications for Design

Designers are encouraged to consider the ecology created from the interactions between all the disciplines involved with autism and the personal experience of the autistic. The place where these must come together and begin is from the bottom, the sensory input. The Experience begins here and therefore very specific user experiences should be designed for before technology aims to work at higher level goals. Understanding how the parts fit together and the potential impact not considering foundational skills could have on end users, the goal of this chapter and of these user experience goals is to highlight the place to begin. to have the greatest impact, designers would not move beyond this level until it's been mastered and adopted and successful across a diverse set of people and platforms. This chapter calls for all Technologies to attempt to mediate sensory sensitivities as a standard design practice details on how to do so occur in the following chapters.

Conclusion

There are key indicators that the gap between what is being built and what is needed by users is increasing. Critical autism studies scholars have called for more work to be done to support sensory and cognitive functioning rather than social behavior which have been perceived as taking away a person's agency (Guberman & Haimson, 2023; Spiel et al., 2019; Williams & Gilbert, 2019) Targeting the outward manifestations of autism are not a

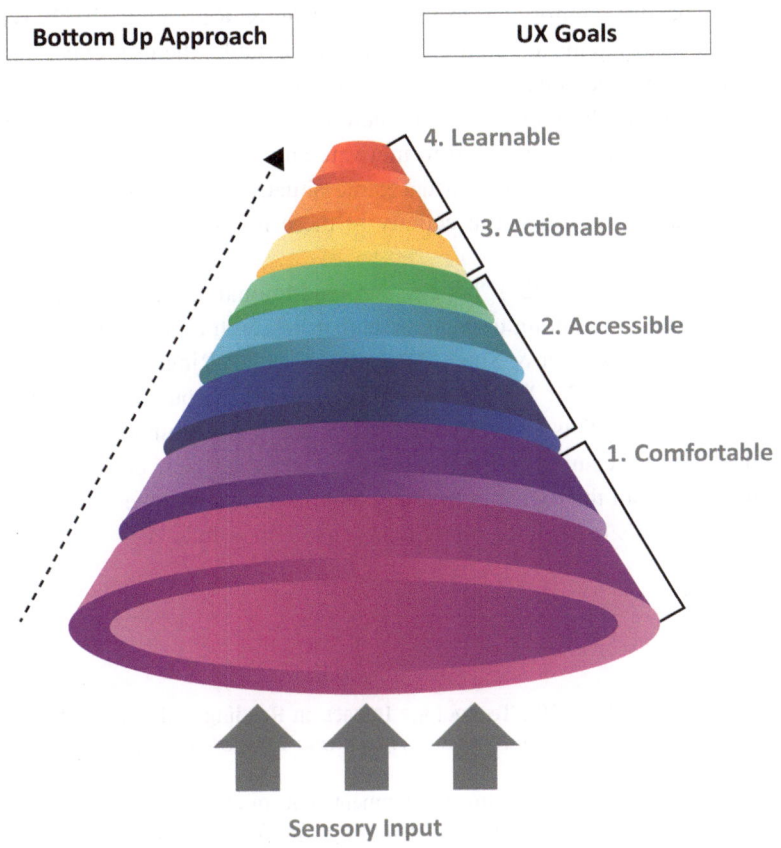

Fig. 2.2 Bottom-up approach with corresponding user experiences goals

priority for this group, rather they are asking for support with internal, invisible processes that dictate the core challenges to daily living. Despite these stated needs, most projects address behaviors, that are high-level skills to achieve observable social skills and communication. These high level processing technologies often do so from a top down model of skill training, omitting the prerequisite, foundational bottom-up information processing challenges that occur at the lower level of sensory processing (Ayres & Robbins, 2005; Bogdashina, 2016; Dunn, 1997; Dunn et al., 2002; Little et al., 2017; Robertson & Baron-Cohen, 2017). In order for these emerging assistive technologies to positively impact one's quality of life, they must first be actionable, accessible, and comfortable (Boyd, 2019), see Fig. 2.2.

Assistive technologies build on evidence from neuroscience and the needs of autistic end users. This research will lay the groundwork for a broader evidence-based and inclusive approach to assistive technologies for a variety of cognitive differences. Operationalize UX goals are to first build a comfortable system. This means the systems are physically and socially comfortable to the user (Deng & Rattadilok, 2022; Williams & Gilbert, 2020). Once systems are comfortable and acceptable, the user experience goal of ensuring information is perceived can be addressed. For example, this Chapter is moving up the rings of skills to the motor section where no motor routines are accessible to the student or previously. These were hard to motivate and make sense. He'd have to do the same motion again and again. In a virtual game situation where he's been made to be comfortable, the action is just a fun activity in there for the practice he needs is now accessible.

Guberman and Haimson (2023) "hope to enroll additional researchers into the growing ranks of HCI scholars attempting to resituate autism research around the wants and needs of autistic *people* (e.g., Kender & Spiel, 2022; Keyes, 2020; Ringland, 2019; Spiel, et al., 2019; Spiel & Gerling, 2021; Williams & Gilbert, 2019; Ymous et al., 2020)" (Guberman & Haimson, 2023). This book proposes the Sensory Accommodation Framework to offer designers a neuro-centric model that bridges a personal-view design where technology is oriented out from the user to improving their experience of the world. This is done by enhancing the user's experience rather than remediating deficits.

References

Abdo, M., & Al Osman, H. (2019). Technology Impact on Reading and writing skills of children with autism: A systematic literature review. *Health and Technology, 9*(5), 725–735. https://doi.org/10.1007/s12553-019-00317-4

Abosi, O., & Koay, T. L. (2008). Attaining development goals of children with disabilities: Implications for inclusive education. *International Journal of Special Education, 23*(3), 1–10.

Accardo, A. L., Finnegan, E. G., Kuder, S. J., & Bomgardner, E. M. (2020). Writing interventions for individuals with autism spectrum disorder: A research synthesis. *Journal of Autism and Developmental Disorders, 50*(6), 1988–2006. https://doi.org/10.1007/s10803-019-03955-9

Apling, R., & Jones, N. L. (2001). *The individuals with disabilities education act (IDEA): Overview of major provisions.* Congressional Research Service, Library of Congress.

Ayres, A. J., & Robbins, J. (2005). *Sensory integration and the child: Understanding hidden sensory challenges.* Western Psychological Services.

Bogdashina, O. (2016). *Sensory perceptual issues in autism and asperger syndrome* (2nd ed.). Jessica Kingsley Publishers.

Boros, M., Anton, J.-L., Pech-Georgel, C., Grainger, J., Szwed, M., & Ziegler, J. C. (2016). *NeuroImage, 128*, 316–327. https://doi.org/10.1016/j.neuroimage.2016.01.014

Boyd, L. (2019). Designing sensory-inclusive virtual play spaces for children. In *Proceedings of the 18th ACM international conference on interaction design and children* (pp. 446–451). https://doi.org/10.1145/3311927.3325315

Boyd, L. E., Gupta, S., Vikmani, S. B., Gutierrez, C. M., Yang, J., Linstead, E., & Hayes, G. R. (2018). vrSocial: Toward immersive therapeutic VR systems for children with autism. In *Proceedings of the 2018 CHI conference on human factors in computing systems* (pp. 1–12). https://doi.org/10.1145/3173574.3173778

Boyd, L. E., Jiang, X., & Hayes, G. R. (2017). ProCom: Designing and evaluating a mobile and wearable system to support proximity awareness for people with autism. In *Proceedings of the*

2017 CHI conference on human factors in computing systems (pp. 2865–2877). https://doi.org/
10.1145/3025453.3026014

Boyd, L. E., Rangel, A., Tomimbang, H., Conejo-Toledo, A., Patel, K., Tentori, M., & Hayes, G. R.
(2016). SayWAT: Augmenting face-to-face conversations for adults with autism. In *Proceedings
of the 2016 CHI conference on human factors in computing systems* (pp. 4872–4883). https://doi.
org/10.1145/2858036.2858215

Boyd, L. E., Ringland, K. E., Haimson, O. L., Fernandez, H., Bistarkey, M., & Hayes, G. R. (2015).
Evaluating a collaborative iPad game's impact on social relationships for children with autism
spectrum disorder. *ACM Transactions on Accessible Computing, 7*(1), 1–18. https://doi.org/10.
1145/2751564

Boyd, L., Garner, E., Kim, I., & Valencia, G. (2022). Cognality VR: Exploring a mobile VR app
with multiple stakeholders to reduce meltdowns in autistic children. In *CHI conference on human
factors in computing systems extended abstracts* (pp. 1–7). https://doi.org/10.1145/3491101.351
9742

Bullen, J. C., Zajic, M. C., McIntyre, N., Solari, E., & Mundy, P. (2022). Patterns of math and reading achievement in children and adolescents with autism spectrum disorder. *Research in Autism
Spectrum Disorders, 92*, 101933. https://doi.org/10.1016/j.rasd.2022.101933

Chez, M. G., Memon, S., & Hung, P. C. (2004). Neurologic treatment strategies in autism: An
overview of medical intervention strategies. *Seminars in Pediatric Neurology, 11*(3), 229–235.
https://doi.org/10.1016/j.spen.2004.07.007

Chiang, H.-M., & Lin, Y.-H. (2007). Mathematical ability of students with Asperger syndrome and
high-functioning autism: A review of literature. *Autism, 11*(6), 547–556. https://doi.org/10.1177/
1362361307083259

Cibrian, F. L., Ley-Flores, J., Newbold, J. W., Singh, A., Bianchi-Berthouze, N., & Tentori, M.
(2021). Interactive sonification to assist children with autism during motor therapeutic interventions. *Personal and Ubiquitous Computing, 25*(2), 391–410. https://doi.org/10.1007/s00779-020-
01479-z

Cibrian, F. L., Peña, O., Ortega, D., & Tentori, M. (2017). BendableSound: An elastic multisensory
surface using touch-based interactions to assist children with severe autism during music therapy.
International Journal of Human-Computer Studies, 107, 22–37. https://doi.org/10.1016/j.ijhcs.
2017.05.003

Del Valle Rubido, M., McCracken, J. T., Hollander, E., Shic, F., Noeldeke, J., Boak, L., Khwaja, O.,
Sadikhov, S., Fontoura, P., & Umbricht, D. (2018). In search of biomarkers for autism spectrum
disorder. *Autism Research, 11*(11), 1567–1579. https://doi.org/10.1002/aur.2026

Deng, L., & Rattadilok, P. (2022). The need for and barriers to using assistive technologies among
individuals with autism spectrum disorders in China. *Assistive Technology, 34*(2), 242–253.
https://doi.org/10.1080/10400435.2020.1757787

DSM History. (n.d.). Retrieved March 14, 2023, from https://www.psychiatry.org:443/psychiatrists/
practice/dsm/about-dsm/history-of-the-dsm

Dunn, W. (1997). The impact of sensory processing abilities on the daily lives of young children
and their families: A conceptual model. *Infants & Young Children, 9*(4), 23–35. https://doi.org/
10.1097/00001163-199704000-00005

Dunn, W., Myles, B. S., & Orr, S. (2002). Sensory processing issues associated with Asperger
syndrome: A preliminary investigation. *American Journal of Occupational Therapy, 56*(1),
97–102.

Escobedo, L., Nguyen, D. H., Boyd, L., Hirano, S., Rangel, A., Garcia-Rosas, D., Tentori, M., &
Hayes, G. (2012). MOSOCO: A mobile assistive tool to support children with autism practicing
social skills in real-life situations. In *Proceedings of the SIGCHI conference on human factors in
computing systems* (pp. 2589–2598).https://doi.org/10.1145/2207676.2208649

Franceschini, S., Bertoni, S., Gianesini, T., Gori, S., & Facoetti, A. (2017). A different vision of dyslexia: Local precedence on global perception. *Scientific Reports, 7*(1), Article 1. https://doi. org/10.1038/s41598-017-17626-1

Goldstein-Marcusohn, Y., Goldfarb, L., & Shany, M. (2020). Global and local visual processing in rate/accuracy subtypes of dyslexia. *Frontiers in Psychology, 11.* https://www.frontiersin.org/art icle/10.3389/fpsyg.2020.00828

Guberman, J., & Haimson, O. (2023). Not robots; Cyborgs—Furthering anti-ableist research in human-computer interaction. *First Monday.* https://doi.org/10.5210/fm.v28i1.12910

Hailpern, J., Karahalios, K., DeThorne, L., & Halle, J. (2010). Vocsyl: Visualizing syllable production for children with ASD and speech delays. In *Proceedings of the 12th international ACM SIGACCESS conference on computers and accessibility* (pp. 297–298). https://doi.org/10.1145/1878803.1878879

Hailpern, J., Karahalios, K., & Halle, J. (2009). Creating a spoken impact: Encouraging vocalization through audio visual feedback in children with ASD. In *Proceedings of the SIGCHI conference on human factors in computing systems* (pp. 453–462).https://doi.org/10.1145/1518701.1518774

Hayes, G. R., & Hosaflook, S. W. (2013). HygieneHelper: Promoting awareness and teaching life skills to youth with autism spectrum disorder. In *Proceedings of the 12th international conference on interaction design and children* (pp. 539–542). https://doi.org/10.1145/2485760.2485860

Henry, J. D., von Hippel, W., Molenberghs, P., Lee, T., & Sachdev, P. S. (2016). Clinical assessment of social cognitive function in neurological disorders. *Nature Reviews Neurology, 12*(1), Article 1. https://doi.org/10.1038/nrneurol.2015.229

Jolliffe, T., & Baron-Cohen, S. (1999). A test of central coherence theory: Linguistic processing in high-functioning adults with autism or Asperger syndrome: Is local coherence impaired? *Cognition, 71*(2), 149–185. https://doi.org/10.1016/S0010-0277(99)00022-0

Kender, K., & Spiel, K. (2022, April). FaceSavr™: Designing technologies with allistic adults to battle emotion echolalia. In CHI Conference on Human Factors in Computing Systems Extended Abstracts (pp. 1-8).

Keyes, O. (2020). Automating autism: Disability, discourse, and artificial intelligence. The Journal of Sociotechnical Critique, 1(1), 8.

Kientz, J. A., Goodwin, M. S., Hayes, G. R., & Abowd, G. D. (2013). Interactive technologies for autism. *Synthesis Lectures on Assistive, Rehabilitative, and Health-Preserving Technologies, 2*(2), 1–177. https://doi.org/10.2200/S00533ED1V01Y201309ARH004

Knight, V., McKissick, B. R., & Saunders, A. (2013). A review of technology-based interventions to teach academic skills to students with autism spectrum disorder. *Journal of Autism and Developmental Disorders, 43*(11), 2628–2648. https://doi.org/10.1007/s10803-013-1814-y

Little, L. M., Dean, E., Tomchek, S., & Dunn, W. (2017). Sensory processing patterns in autism, attention deficit hyperactivity disorder, and typical development. *Physical & Occupational Therapy in Pediatrics*, 1–12. https://doi.org/10.1080/01942638.2017.1390809

Madsen, M., el Kaliouby, R., Goodwin, M., & Picard, R. (2008). Technology for just-in-time in-situ learning of facial affect for persons diagnosed with an autism spectrum disorder. In *Proceedings of the 10th international ACM SIGACCESS conference on computers and accessibility* (pp. 19–26). https://doi.org/10.1145/1414471.1414477

Martin, E. W., Martin, R., & Terman, D. L. (1996). The legislative and litigation history of special education. *The Future of Children, 6*(1), 25–39. https://doi.org/10.2307/1602492

Monarca, I., Chen, Y. Y., Bichelmeir, A., Anderson, K., Tentori, M., & Cibrian, F. L. (2023). Designing a game for haptic interfaces to uncover gestural pattern in children. In J. Bravo, S. Ochoa, & J. Favela (Eds.), *Proceedings of the international conference on ubiquitous computing & ambient intelligence (UCAmI 2022)* (pp. 944–948). Springer International Publishing. https://doi.org/10.1007/978-3-031-21333-5_93

Monarca, I., Tentori, M., & Cibrian, F. L. (2021). Feel and touch: A haptic mobile game to assess tactile processing. *Avances En Interacción Humano-Computadora, 1,* 31. https://doi.org/10.47756/aihc.y6i1.83

Parés, N., Carreras, A., Durany, J., Ferrer, J., Freixa, P., Gómez, D., Kruglanski, O., Parés, R., Ribas, J. I., Soler, M., & Sanjurjo, À. (n.d.). *MEDIATE: An interactive multisensory environment for children with severe autism and no verbal communication.*

Pennington, M. L., Cullinan, D., & Southern, L. B. (2014). Defining autism: Variability in state education agency definitions of and evaluations for autism spectrum disorders. *Autism Research and Treatment, 2014,* 327271. https://doi.org/10.1155/2014/327271

Piper, A. M., O'Brien, E., Morris, M. R., & Winograd, T. (2006). SIDES: A cooperative tabletop computer game for social skills development. In *Proceedings of the 2006 20th anniversary conference on computer supported cooperative work* (pp. 1–10). https://doi.org/10.1145/1180875.1180877

Pollind, M., Soangra, R., Grant-Beuttler, M., & Aminian, A. (2019). Customized wearable sensor-based insoles for gait re-training in idiopathic toe walkers. *Biomedical Sciences Instrumentation, 55*(2), 192–198.

Prior, M. R., & Hall, L. C. (1979). Comprehension of transitive and intransitive phrases by autistic, retarded, and normal children. *Journal of Communication Disorders, 12*(2), 103–111. https://doi.org/10.1016/0021-9924(79)90033-9

Ramachandiran, C. R., Jomhari, N., Thiyagaraja, S., & Maria, M. (2015). Virtual reality based behavioral learning for autistic children. *Electronic Journal of E-Learning, 13*(5), Article 5.

Rapp, A., Cena, F., Castaldo, R., Keller, R., & Tirassa, M. (2018). Designing technology for spatial needs: Routines, control and social competences of people with autism. *International Journal of Human-Computer Studies, 120,* 49–65. https://doi.org/10.1016/j.ijhcs.2018.07.005

Rello, L., & Baeza-Yates, R. (2016). The effect of font type on screen readability by people with dyslexia. *ACM Transactions on Accessible Computing, 8*(4), 1–33. https://doi.org/10.1145/2897736

Rello, L., & Bigham, J. P. (2017). Good background colors for readers: A study of people with and without dyslexia. In *Proceedings of the 19th international ACM SIGACCESS conference on computers and accessibility* (pp. 72–80). https://doi.org/10.1145/3132525.3132546

Ringland, K. E., Zalapa, R., Neal, M., Escobedo, L., Tentori, M., & Hayes, G. R. (2014). *SensoryPaint: A multimodal sensory intervention for children with neurodevelopmental disorders* (pp. 873–884). https://doi.org/10.1145/2632048.2632065

Ringland, K. E. (2019). "Autsome": Fostering an Autistic Identity in an Online Minecraft Community for Youth with Autism. In Information in Contemporary Society: 14th International Conference, iConference 2019, Washington, DC, USA, March 31–April 3, 2019, Proceedings 14 (pp. 132-143). Springer International Publishing.

Robertson, C. E., & Baron-Cohen, S. (2017). Sensory perception in autism. *Nature Reviews Neuroscience, 18*(11), 671–684. https://doi.org/10.1038/nrn.2017.112

Simm, W., Ferrario, M. A., Gradinar, A., & Whittle, J. (2014). Prototyping "clasp": Implications for designing digital technology for and with adults with autism. In *Proceedings of the 2014 conference on designing interactive systems* (pp. 345–354). https://doi.org/10.1145/2598510.2600880

Spiel, K., Frauenberger, C., Keyes, O., & Fitzpatrick, G. (2019). Agency of autistic children in technology research: A critical literature review. *ACM Transactions on Computer-Human Interaction, 26*(6), 38:1–38:40. https://doi.org/10.1145/3344919

Spiel, K., & Gerling, K. (2021). The purpose of play: How HCI games research fails neurodivergent populations. ACM Transactions on Computer-Human Interaction (TOCHI), 28(2), 1–40.

Stein, J. (2014). Dyslexia: The role of vision and visual attention. *Current Developmental Disorders Reports, 1*(4), 267–280. https://doi.org/10.1007/s40474-014-0030-6

Takahashi, I., Oki, M., Bourreau, B., Kitahara, I., & Suzuki, K. (2018). FUTUREGYM: A gymnasium with interactive floor projection for children with special needs. *International Journal of Child-Computer Interaction, 15*, 37–47. https://doi.org/10.1016/j.ijcci.2017.12.002

Tsermentseli, S., O'Brien, J. M., & Spencer, J. V. (2008). Comparison of form and motion coherence processing in autistic spectrum disorders and dyslexia. *Journal of Autism and Developmental Disorders, 38*(7), 1201–1210. https://doi.org/10.1007/s10803-007-0500-3

Ulgado, R. R., Nguyen, K., Custodio, V. E., Waterhouse, A., Weiner, R., & Hayes, G. (2013). VidCoach: A mobile video modeling system for youth with special needs. In *Proceedings of the 12th international conference on interaction design and children* (pp. 581–584). https://doi.org/10.1145/2485760.2485870

Vidyasagar, T. R. (2004). Neural underpinnings of dyslexia as a disorder of visuo-spatial attention. *Clinical and Experimental Optometry, 87*(1), 4–10. https://doi.org/10.1111/j.1444-0938.2004.tb03138.x

Washington, P., Voss, C., Kline, A., Haber, N., Daniels, J., Fazel, A., De, T., Feinstein, C., Winograd, T., & Wall, D. (2017). SuperpowerGlass: A wearable aid for the at-home therapy of children with autism. In *Proceedings of the ACM on interactive, mobile, wearable and ubiquitous technologies* (vol. 1(3), pp. 112:1–112:22). https://doi.org/10.1145/3130977

Williams, R. M., & Gilbert, J. E. (2019). Cyborg perspectives on computing research reform. In *Extended abstracts of the 2019 CHI conference on human factors in computing systems* (pp. 1–11). https://doi.org/10.1145/3290607.3310421

Williams, R. M., & Gilbert, J. E. (2020). Perseverations of the academy: A survey of wearable technologies applied to autism intervention. *International Journal of Human-Computer Studies, 143*, 102485. https://doi.org/10.1016/j.ijhcs.2020.102485

Yan, Z., Wu, Y., Zhang, Y., & Chen, X. "Anthony." (2022). EmoGlass: An end-to-end AI-enabled wearable platform for enhancing self-awareness of emotional health. In *CHI conference on human factors in computing systems* (pp. 1–19). https://doi.org/10.1145/3491102.3501925

Ymous, A., Spiel, K., Keyes, O., Williams, R. M., Good, J., Hornecker, E., & Bennett, C. L. (2020, April). "I am just terrified of my future"—Epistemic Violence in Disability Related Technology Research. In Extended Abstracts of the 2020 CHI Conference on Human Factors in Computing Systems (pp. 1–16).

Zeidan, J., Fombonne, E., Scorah, J., Ibrahim, A., Durkin, M. S., Saxena, S., Yusuf, A., Shih, A., & Elsabbagh, M. (2022). Global prevalence of autism: A systematic review update. *Autism Research, 15*(5), 778–790. https://doi.org/10.1002/aur.2696

Zolyomi, A., Ross, A. S., Bhattacharya, A., Milne, L., & Munson, S. A. (2018). Values, identity, and social translucence: Neurodiverse student teams in higher education. In *Proceedings of the 2018 CHI conference on human factors in computing systems* (pp. 1–13). https://doi.org/10.1145/3173574.3174073

Sensory Processing in Autism

Sensory Perception

Assistive technology has a long tradition of employing a user's strengths regarding their sensory profile to work around the user's sensory impairments (Dunn, 2014). Some of the ways researchers and commercial products have explored integrating dominant sensory modalities to support non-dominant sensory modalities into computational systems depending on the persons, individual strength, as well as the nature of the task. Other technologies address developing foundational skills such as coordinating body movements and self-regulation.

Auditory Processing

Auditory processing is the ability to hear sounds, differentiate between different sounds, make meaning from sounds, and selectively tune into or tune out certain sounds (Audiologist, 2022; International, 2015; Selinger, n.d.). It is the processing of sound beyond simply hearing which is the sound being received by the ear. The processing that occurs after the sound signals are received occurs in the brain. Auditory processing makes sense of the sounds as speech or nonspeech. Listening comprehension however is a higher level of processing that makes sense of the speech sounds (Selinger, n.d.). Auditory channels provide a powerful alternative to visual perception (Guerreiro & Gonçalves, 2014). Autistic children have demonstrated a hypersensitivity to sound as demonstrated in as compared to typically developing children in the auditory domain, as "auditory processing items primarily reflect sensitivity (i.e., 'Is distracted when there is a lot of noise around', 'holds hands over ears to protect them from sound')" (Little et al., 2017). Additionally, researchers have found that autistic people can be hyposensitive to audio input, may seek out loud sounds, or have difficulty tuning into language (International, 2015) (see sensory patterns and profiles in the next chapter).

Hearing is a strength for some disabled people and has been used in multiple assistive technology systems (Ratanasit & Moore, 2005). The pervasive use of audio results from the relative ease of preparing information designed for other channels. For example, descriptions of visual elements (e.g., color, emphasis, and spatial arrangement) provide textual information of visualizations. There are standards to support this translation (Reid & Snow-Weaver, 2008). Complex information communicated auditorily is delivered serially. Audio's serial and ephemeral nature limits the rate and expressiveness of audio information. Once auditory stimuli is presented, it is then gone. Without intervention, the stimuli is unretrievable. To counter the dissipating temporal nature of audio, researchers have leveraged the human ability to process sounds in three dimensions through 3D (Daft & Lengel, 1986) as well as concurrent speech (Guerreiro & Gonçalves, 2014). These approaches are particularly well suited for users who have significantly stronger verbal auditory encoding abilities (Röder et al., 2001).

Tactile Processing

Tactile processing is the process of detecting of and discriminating information via touch. The sense of touch includes light touch, deep pressure, vibration, and temperature (*Tactile Processing, Part 1*, n.d.). The sense of touch is a rich input modality. It can perceive a diverse range of feedback from size and shape to texture, stiffness, and temperature (Klatzky & Lederman, 2003). The richness of the tactile modality makes it suitable for a variety of assistive tasks. For example, augmenting visual memorization tasks with tactile cues is an effective memory aid for individuals with poor recall abilities (Kuznetsov et al., 2009). However, people with autism have demonstrated hypo and hyper sensitivity to tactile input (Tavassoli et al., 2016), although research on this phenomenon is mixed in terms of finding evidence and a neurobiological root (Mikkelsen et al., 2018).

Technologies that aim to support the integration of tactile stimuli. Bendable sound is a multi-sensory system using a large-scale elastic display enabling autistic children to play with sounds when practicing coordinating movements such as tapping, pushing or pinching. Bendable sound includes musical notes arranged in an ascendant way and the 3D animated Neon background of space nebulas with translucent space elements such as rockets and planets. Bendable sound is open-ended and structured activities with challenges related to rhythm and strength (Cibrian et al., 2017; Monica et al., 2023a, 2023b). One project uses touch as part of the solution aimed at, Clasp was designed to alleviate anxiety with adults with autism by delivering tactile input to learn about anxiety-producing events (Simm et al., 2014).

Proprioception Processing

Proprioception is the sense of body awareness regarding movement, force of movement, position and posture of the body (Balasubramanian & Santos, 2014). Individuals with sensory deficits in this area may lack awareness of certain body parts and how those parts move. Proprioception sensors are located within the muscles and joints and are activated when the muscle contracts (Myles et al., 2001). Proprioception is a relatively underutilized form of digital communication; proprioception offers promising new paradigms for controlling information flow to and from computing systems.

Researchers have explored incorporating proprioception into computational systems through gestural control (Folmer & Morelli, 2012; Lopes et al., 2015), on-body interfaces (Folmer & Morelli, 2012; Harrison et al., 2010; Yu & Brewster, 2003), and physical environments (Oh & Findlater, 2015). Although proprioceptive accuracy has been shown to vary across ability (Ament et al., 2015) and age (Adamo et al., 2007), the differences are not significant enough to preclude it as a tool for interaction (Oh & Findlater, 2015). To increase the richness of input, proprioception is frequently used in combination with tactile input (Li et al., 2010). For example, Folmer and Morelli's system used vibrotactile feedback and gestural arm movements, providing a bi-directional control environment through which the system can respond to the input from the user and vice versa (Folmer & Morelli, 2012). Similarly, Li et al., report an 83% accuracy rate by visually impaired participants using mobile phone sensors to locate virtual objects in a 3D space (Li et al., 2010).

In autism research, proprioception has been described by researchers as hypersensitivity in some cases where children displayed problems such as toe walking. Alternatively, people may be hypo-sensitive where they engage in purposely crashing their body into objects or falling behavior as well as difficulty planning motor sequences (Blanche et al., 2012). To address proprioception-seeking, a digital hugging vest was explicitly designed to support supplying deep pressure touch on demand for autistic children (Duvall et al., 2016). Lastly, haptic interfaces have provided a comfortable experience as well as clinical information of the physical effort or strength of the touch, an important developmental skill, exhibited by the child (Monica et al., 2023a, 2023b).

Interoception

Interoception is the ability to interpret one's own bodily sensations such as respiration, hunger, heartbeat, need to urinate, and pain. Interoception is perceived through the receptors in the skin as well as internal organs. This sensory system related to pain perception has been described as hypo or hypersensitive in autistic people, although not in statically significant ways (Williams et al., 2023). In the case of hyposensitivity, a person with autism can get hurt from not feeling the sensation of pain, for example a person with autism may be overly sensitive to or under sensitive the temperature of bath water (Shah, 2016). In the case of hypersensitivity to internal indications, researchers hypothesize that "heightened attention to internal cues may lead to decreased attention to external stimuli, which provides a putative link between decreased social interaction and repetitive patterns of behavior that directs the focus of attention inward" (Schauder et al., 2015). Therefore, gaining the user's attention to sensory input originating from outside one's body needs to occur before someone can process the information.

Visual Processing

Visual processing is the main sensory system with almost 80% of the cortex dedicated to visual processing (Kafaligonul, 2014). Visual processing generally is a well-known strength in autism research (Mottron et al., 2006; Myles, 2001; Robertson & Baron-Cohen, 2017). Several assistive technology projects have leveraged this strength in technologies for autism. For example, MOSOCO (Escobedo et al., 2012) is a mobile app that steps through visual steps of social interaction. vSked (Hirano et al., 2010) is an interactive visual schedule used in specialized classrooms for autistic children. SIDES (Piper et al., 2006) was developed after researchers observed that autistic children prefer visual games. They followed this preference with a "highly visual four player game" to support collaboration skills using a tabletop surface. For larger group collaboration, Future gym visualizes cues on the gymnasium floor for autistic children to follow step by step routines and games (Takahashi et al., 2018).

The Spoken Impact project (Hailpern et al., 2009) and VocSyl (Hailpern et al., 2010) employed visualization of speech sounds and utterance length to promote vocalizations in autistic children. SensoryPaint (Ringland et al., 2014) provides a whole body interaction with a Kinect system and results in a wall-sized visualization of children's movements (or results of their movements in the form of a digital imprint where a physical ball they threw hit the wall.

Filtering out information to support visual processing is also a common strategy in technology for autism. To support social skills and mediate sensory challenges for people with autism, Parson leverages filtering out of much of the face to face stimulation that occurs when users interact in VR (Parsons, 2000). Her research spans from Virtual Reality on desktops to more advanced virtual reality systems with avatars (Parsons & Cobb, 2011; Parsons et al., 2006). These related works offer a range of possibilities for providing alternative input to the user based on form through sensory strengths. These support an alternative **form** of information, but do not necessarily explicitly provide information on the **structure** or function of the information, communicated through different sensory channels that independently play a role in processing (Grinter et al., 2010).

Global and Local Visual Processing

The overall structure of information is communicated through the gist derived the global information that is processed in the dorsal stream of the brain, an area indicated as involved with a number of developmental disorders (Atkinson, 2017; Chen et al., 2019; Doniger et al., 2002; Grinter et al., 2010; Sonuga-Barke & Fairchild, 2012).

These two streams are integrated over time. This process is most obvious when stimuli are continuously processed rather than viewing static information (Ito et al., 2017; Kojovic et al., 2020). Technologies that support visual support for dyslexia have adjusted background colors (Rello & Bigham, 2017) and fonts (Rello & Baeza-Yates, 2016). Attention to text, photos, and symbols has been examined to provide simplified information for autistic children (Yaneva et al., 2015), and Phonoblocks has utilized color coding for contextual spelling rules for dyslexia (Cramer et al., 2016).

Regarding global–local visual processing for autism, spatial frequency has been manipulated to mimic a global precedence (Boyd et al., 2022) as autistic participants have been found to respond differently to high and low spatial frequency (de Jong et al., 2008; Deruelle et al., 2004; Hübner, 1997). Explicit intervention for these differences has been explored by intervention (Boyd et al., 2022). Luminance and Chroma have also been manipulated to model a global–local progression via filtering images before stimulus presentation (Sean, 2020).

It is clear that new technologies must address one of the hidden challenges in autism: the inefficient integration of multiple sensory channels caused by local interference. Local interference occurs when prioritizing local details derails complete processing of information. One must comprehend the overall structure of information (global information) to understand the 'gist'. Local interference halts global processing, the autistic individual is left with a highly detailed, but contextually disconnected perception of their situation. Global precedence is often assumed to be the primary style (Baumann & Kuhl, 2005). However, this is not the case for many people as several factors impact global or local precedence. For example, when observing a forest, an assemblage of trees, the observer has all the information to take in but which system is activated first—is it the whole scene or narrowed focus on details? One's precedence can be affected by the task type and attention, so in neurocognitive science research, contrived stimuli and tasks are created to discern one's precedence. See Chap. 5 for general system design strategies for global processing, Chap. 6 for social cognition related to global processing's role in visual attention.

Vestibular

This is the sense of orientation and direction that is detected in the inner ear canals. The vestibular system is another component of the sensory systems that helps individuals with their sense of balance. This system "provides information about where our body is in space, and whether we or our surroundings are moving. The vestibular system also informs the body about speed and direction of movement," (Myles et al., 2000, p. 5). This system is regulated by the inner ear, and it is "stimulated by head movements and input from other senses," (Myles et al., 2000, p. 5). For individuals who are medically fragile or have vestibular deficits that would make it too risky for them to be part of the outside world, a virtual reality system provides users with real-world experiences (Viirre et al., 2001). For autistic children in movement therapy, Dancecraft was created to provide a visualization of one's dance performance captured by a video game console with wireless motion sensing and gesture recognition (Ringland et al., 2019).

Olfactory Processing

The olfactory system provides information to the brain about the smells in the environment. This powerful system can trigger memories and allows individuals to embed learning through the sense of smell. Chemical receptors are located in the nasal structure and react to the smells in the environment (Myles et al., 2000; Robertson & Baron-Cohen, 2017). For individuals with hypersensitivity to smell (i.e., perfume) may prefer to participate in everyday outside activities and VR may be a necessary tool for learning in a contained environment. On the hyposensitivity end of the olfactory processing spectrum someone with a difficulty making decisions based on smell may benefit from a technology that can smell for them; one such project was explored where sensors were developed to determine cooking states and food for novice cooks (Hirano, 2016).

Sensory Differences as Design Requirements

Given the complexity of sensory processing, the use of sensory patterns is helpful to technology designers as a lens to accommodate universal wants and needs. Sensory wants and needs are user requirements. From a *sensory-first approach*, a designer first addresses sensory preferences before designing social or functional skill supports. This is particularly important because conditions such as autism have been traditionally supported by assistive technologies aimed to correct atypical behavior, teach skills, identify, or prompt the identification of aspects of the environment (e.g., emotions of others)—thus addressing only the behavioral and cognitive aspects of the condition. Few to none have explicitly considered the core challenge of sensory processing. Most environments are designed for typical sensory processing, underscoring the validity of the social model of disability and need to design technology with a sensory perspective.

Sensory processing patterns and challenges impact activities of daily living not only for autistic people (Ayres & Robbins, 2005; Bogdashina, 2016; Dunn, 1997; Dunn et al., 2002; Robertson & Baron-Cohen, 2017; Roley et al., 2014) but also those with ADHD

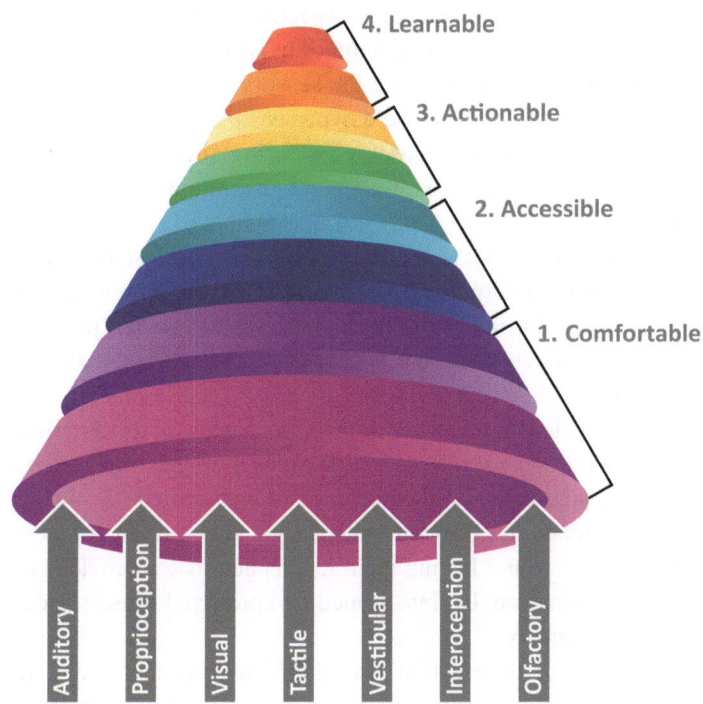

Fig. 3.1 Sensory-first approach with user experience goals of making technology comfortable, accessible, actionable, and learnable

(Little et al., 2017; Schulze et al., 2020, 2021), and dyslexia (Ali et al., 2021; Formoso et al., 2022a, 2022b; Franceschini et al., 2017; Goldstein-Marcusohn et al., 2020; Liu et al., 2022). Therefore, the prioritization of the customizable sensory input and output in the design of technology as approximately 15% of the USA population is suspected to live with sensory processing disorders (Galiana-Simal et al., 2020). Therefore, understanding the unique profiles of individual users as well as communities of users is paramount to building a comfortable and useful technology (Fig. 3.1).

Implications for Design

How to apply these sensory profiles to system design patterns is discussed in detail in the following chapters (Dunn, 2014). Overall, the goals are to ensure that sensory input and sensory environments are customizable so that the user can be comfortable in the environment, access the information provided by the system, act upon the information provided by the system, and learn from the system. The following general design implication are discussed further in the subsequent chapters:

1. Allow for reduction or increase of channel-specific sensory input. Autistic people and those with sensory sensitivities can be hypo or hypersensitive to any sensory modality thus, there is an opportunity to mediate the sensory experience to free up processing resources. For example, if someone were hypersensitive to tactile input, such that they Wish to avoid putting on a VR headset, considering alternative form factors or platforms that do not require touch would allow the user to put their reserved energy into the experience.

2. Split or condense information into separate channels or collapse into one. For example, if someone has difficulty interpreting the tone of voice, separating out the literal meaning of the words from the intended meaning conveyed through procity into separate streams of information can allow the person to access the nonverbal communication they may miss when it's presented orally.

3. Allowing for varying levels of automation or user control for user interactions. For example, if someone has sensory motor difficulties they may prefer certain user interactions to be automated to allow for higher level engagement. In the case of playing video games, if someone has difficulty using a game controller but very much wants to engage in the social banter having their actions automated provides entry into play.

4. Allow for sensory channels to be transformed into preferred sensory modalities or even single modality (unisensory).

5. Allow for recapturing of information "freezing" the screen or audio stream to allow for a customizable window of time to process. For example, if someone has difficulty monitoring how much time has passed while they're also talking to someone, providing a visual persistent representation of time passing, can ease the burden of integrating temporal information.

6. Capture key moments of information and provide customizable playback speed. For example, if someone is reading closed captions while viewing a movie, allow for the playback speed to be paused or slowed down on demand to allow for time to process the written word with the on-screen action.

7. Augment information that may not be perceivable such as facial expression. For example, if someone is using a strategy of looking away from a person while they speak to focus on the auditory channel of what they're saying, they may miss facial expressions that go along with what they're saying. Augmenting facial expressions using additional information presented through a system could capture some of the missing information.

These design principles are explored in more detail in Chaps. 4 through 7.

Conclusion

Although people with sensory processing differences may incorporate multiple sensory channels or switch between channels to understand and navigate through the world, technology design may not represent or differentiate levels or both types of information streams for all modalities. These implications are general guidelines to improve the comfort, accessibility/perceivable, actionability, and learning of information provided by assistive and accessibility technologies for autism.

References

Adamo, D. E., Martin, B. J., & Brown, S. H. (2007). Age-related differences in upper limb proprioceptive acuity. *Perceptual and Motor Skills, 104*(3_suppl), 1297–1309. https://doi.org/10.2466/pms.104.4.1297-1309

Ali, S. A., Fadzil, N. A., Reza, F., Mustafar, F., & Begum, T. (2021). A mini review: Visual and auditory perception in Dyslexia. *IIUM Medical Journal Malaysia, 20*(4), Article 4. https://doi.org/10.31436/imjm.v20i4.1616

Ament, K., Mejia, A., Buhlman, R., Erklin, S., Caffo, B., Mostofsky, S., & Wodka, E. (2015). Evidence for specificity of motor impairments in catching and balance in children with autism. *Journal of Autism and Developmental Disorders, 45*(3), 742–751. https://doi.org/10.1007/s10803-014-2229-0

Atkinson, J. (2017). The Davida teller award lecture, 2016: Visual brain development: A review of "Dorsal Stream Vulnerability"—motion, mathematics, amblyopia, actions, and attention. *Journal of Vision, 17*(3), 26. https://doi.org/10.1167/17.3.26

Audiologist, D. K. L. K. (2022, December 7). *What Is central auditory processing disorder? | Denton hearing.* https://dentonhearing.com/patient-resources/what-is-central-auditory-processing-disorder/

Ayres, A. J., & Robbins, J. (2005). *Sensory integration and the child: Understanding hidden sensory challenges.* Western Psychological Services.

Balasubramanian, R., & Santos, V. J. (2014). *The human hand as an inspiration for robot hand development.* Springer.

Baumann, N., & Kuhl, J. (2005). Positive affect and flexibility: Overcoming the precedence of global over local processing of visual information. *Motivation and Emotion, 29*(2), 123–134. https://doi.org/10.1007/s11031-005-7957-1

Blanche, E. I., Reinoso, G., Chang, M. C., & Bodison, S. (2012). Proprioceptive processing difficulties among children with autism spectrum disorders and developmental disabilities. *The American Journal of Occupational Therapy, 66*(5), 621–624. https://doi.org/10.5014/ajot.2012.004234

Bogdashina, O. (2016). *Sensory perceptual issues in autism and asperger syndrome* (2nd ed.). Jessica Kingsley Publishers.

Boyd, L., Berardi, V., Hughes, D., Cibrian, F., Johnson, J., Sean, V., DelPizzo-Cheng, E., Mackin, B., Tusneem, A., Mody, R., Jones, S., & Lotich, K. (2022). Manipulating image luminance to improve eye gaze and verbal behavior in autistic children. *Humanities and Social Sciences Communications, 9*(1), Article 1. https://doi.org/10.1057/s41599-022-01131-6

Chen, H., Liu, K., Zhang, B., Zhang, J., Xue, X., Lin, Y., Zou, D., Chen, M., Kong, Y., Wen, G., Yan, J., & Deng, Y. (2019). More optimal but less regulated dorsal and ventral visual networks in patients with major depressive disorder. *Journal of Psychiatric Research, 110*, 172–178. https://doi.org/10.1016/j.jpsychires.2019.01.005

Cibrian, F. L., Peña, O., Ortega, D., & Tentori, M. (2017). BendableSound: An elastic multisensory surface using touch-based interactions to assist children with severe autism during music therapy. *International Journal of Human-Computer Studies, 107*, 22–37. https://doi.org/10.1016/j.ijhcs.2017.05.003

Cramer, E. S., Antle, A. N., & Fan, M. (2016). The code of many colours: Evaluating the effects of a dynamic colour-coding scheme on children's spelling in a tangible software system. In *Proceedings of the 15th International Conference on Interaction Design and Children* (pp. 473–485). https://doi.org/10.1145/2930674.2930692

Daft, R. L., & Lengel, R. H. (1986). Organizational information requirements, media richness and structural design. *Management Science, 32*(5), 554–571.

de Jong, M. C., van Engeland, H., & Kemner, C. (2008). Attentional effects of gaze shifts are influenced by emotion and spatial frequency, but not in autism. *Journal of the American Academy of Child & Adolescent Psychiatry, 47*(4), 443–454. https://doi.org/10.1097/CHI.0b013e31816429a6

Deruelle, C., Rondan, C., Gepner, B., & Tardif, C. (2004). Spatial frequency and face processing in children with autism and asperger syndrome. *Journal of Autism and Developmental Disorders, 34*(2), 199–210. https://doi.org/10.1023/B:JADD.0000022610.09668.4c

Doniger, G. M., Foxe, J. J., Murray, M. M., Higgins, B. A., & Javitt, D. C. (2002). Impaired visual object recognition and dorsal/ventral stream interaction in schizophrenia. *Archives of General Psychiatry, 59*(11), 1011–1020. https://doi.org/10.1001/archpsyc.59.11.1011

Dunn, W. (1997). The impact of sensory processing abilities on the daily lives of young children and their families: A conceptual model. *Infants & Young Children, 9*(4), 23–35. https://doi.org/10.1097/00001163-199704000-00005

Dunn, W. (2014). *Sensory Profile^{TM} 2*. Pearson.

Dunn, W., Myles, B. S., & Orr, S. (2002). Sensory processing issues associated with Asperger syndrome: A preliminary investigation. *American Journal of Occupational Therapy, 56*(1), 97–102.

Duvall, J. C., Dunne, L. E., Schleif, N., & Holschuh, B. (2016). Active "hugging" vest for deep touch pressure therapy. In *Proceedings of the 2016 ACM international joint conference on pervasive and ubiquitous computing: Adjunct* (pp. 458–463). https://doi.org/10.1145/2968219.2971344

Escobedo, L., Nguyen, D. H., Boyd, L., Hirano, S., Rangel, A., Garcia-Rosas, D., Tentori, M., & Hayes, G. (2012). MOSOCO: A mobile assistive tool to support children with autism practicing social skills in real-life situations. In *Proceedings of the SIGCHI conference on human factors in computing systems* (pp. 2589–2598). https://doi.org/10.1145/2207676.2208649

Folmer, E., & Morelli, T. (2012). *Spatial gestures using a tactile-proprioceptive display, 139*. https://doi.org/10.1145/2148131.2148161

Formoso, M. A., Ortiz, A., Martínez-Murcia, F. J., Brítez, D. A., Escobar, J. J., & Luque, J. L. (2022a). Temporal phase synchrony disruption in dyslexia: Anomaly patterns in auditory processing. In J. M. Ferrández Vicente, J. R. Álvarez-Sánchez, F. de la Paz López, & H. Adeli (Eds.), *Artificial intelligence in neuroscience: Affective analysis and health applications* (Vol. 13258, pp. 13–22). Springer International Publishing. https://doi.org/10.1007/978-3-031-06242-1_2

Formoso, M. A., Ortiz, A., Martínez-Murcia, F. J., Brítez, D. A., Escobar, J. J., & Luque, J. L. (2022b). Temporal phase synchrony disruption in dyslexia: Anomaly patterns in auditory processing. In J. M. Ferrández Vicente, J. R. Álvarez-Sánchez, F. de la Paz López, & H. Adeli (Eds.),

Artificial intelligence in neuroscience: Affective analysis and health applications (Vol. 13258, pp. 13–22). Springer International Publishing. https://doi.org/10.1007/978-3-031-06242-1_2

Franceschini, S., Bertoni, S., Gianesini, T., Gori, S., & Facoetti, A. (2017). A different vision of dyslexia: Local precedence on global perception. *Scientific Reports, 7*(1), Article 1. https://doi.org/10.1038/s41598-017-17626-1

Galiana-Simal, A., Vela-Romero, M., Romero-Vela, V. M., Oliver-Tercero, N., García-Olmo, V., Benito-Castellanos, P. J., Muñoz-Martinez, V., & Beato-Fernandez, L. (2020). Sensory processing disorder: Key points of a frequent alteration in neurodevelopmental disorders. *Cogent Medicine, 7*(1). https://doi.org/10.1080/2331205X.2020.1736829

Goldstein-Marcusohn, Y., Goldfarb, L., & Shany, M. (2020). Global and local visual processing in rate/accuracy subtypes of Dyslexia. *Frontiers in Psychology, 11*. https://www.frontiersin.org/article/10.3389/fpsyg.2020.00828

Grinter, E. J., Maybery, M. T., & Badcock, D. R. (2010). Vision in developmental disorders: Is there a dorsal stream deficit? *Brain Research Bulletin, 82*(3), 147–160. https://doi.org/10.1016/j.brainresbull.2010.02.016

Guerreiro, J., & Gonçalves, D. (2014). Text-to-speeches: Evaluating the perception of concurrent speech by blind people. In *Proceedings of the 16th international ACM SIGACCESS conference on computers & accessibility* (pp. 169–176). https://doi.org/10.1145/2661334.2661367

Hailpern, J., Karahalios, K., DeThorne, L., & Halle, J. (2010). Vocsyl: Visualizing syllable production for children with ASD and speech delays. In *Proceedings of the 12th international ACM SIGACCESS conference on computers and accessibility* (pp. 297–298). https://doi.org/10.1145/1878803.1878879

Hailpern, J., Karahalios, K., & Halle, J. (2009). Creating a spoken impact: Encouraging vocalization through audio visual feedback in children with ASD. In *Proceedings of the SIGCHI conference on human factors in computing systems* (pp. 453–462).https://doi.org/10.1145/1518701.1518774

Harrison, C., Tan, D., & Morris, D. (2010). Skinput: Appropriating the body as an input surface. In *Proceedings of the SIGCHI conference on human factors in computing systems* (pp. 453–462).

Hirano, S. H. (2016). *Designing and evaluating novel interactive technologies using gas sensors to support novice cooks* [Ph.D., University of California, Irvine]. https://www.proquest.com/docview/1886116254/abstract/ECD2A36FF69F4D52PQ/1

Hirano, S. H., Yeganyan, M. T., Marcu, G., Nguyen, D. H., Boyd, L. A., & Hayes, G. R. (2010). vSked: Evaluation of a system to support classroom activities for children with autism. In *Proceedings of the SIGCHI conference on human factors in computing systems* (pp. 1633–1642). https://doi.org/10.1145/1753326.1753569

Hübner, R. (1997). The effect of spatial frequency on global precedence and hemispheric differences. *Perception & Psychophysics, 59*(2), 187–201.

International, N. (2015, August 20). *Auditory Processing—What is It? (Hearing vs. Processing).* NACD International | The National Association for Child Development. https://www.nacd.org/auditory-processing-what-is-it-hearing-vs-processing/

Ito, J., Yamane, Y., Suzuki, M., Maldonado, P., Fujita, I., Tamura, H., & Grün, S. (2017). Switch from ambient to focal processing mode explains the dynamics of free viewing eye movements. *Scientific Reports, 7*(1), Article 1. https://doi.org/10.1038/s41598-017-01076-w

Kafaligonul, H. (2014). *Vision: A systems neuroscience perspective.* http://earsiv.uskudar.edu.tr/xmlui/handle/20.500.12526/535

Klatzky, R. L., & Lederman, S. J. (2003). *Sensory aspects of touch* (Vol. 4).

Kojovic, N., Franchini, M., Sperdin, H. F., Sandini, C., Jan, R. K., Zöller, D., & Schaer, M. (2020). Unraveling the developmental dynamic of visual exploration of social interactions in autism [Preprint]. *Neuroscience.* https://doi.org/10.1101/2020.09.14.290106

Kuznetsov, S., Dey, A. K., & Hudson, S. E. (2009). The effectiveness of haptic cues as an assistive technology for human memory. In H. Tokuda, M. Beigl, A. Friday, A. J. B. Brush, & Y. Tobe (Eds.), *Pervasive computing* (pp. 168–175). Springer. https://doi.org/10.1007/978-3-642-01516-8_12

Li, F. C. Y., Dearman, D., & Truong, K. N. (2010). Leveraging proprioception to make mobile phones more accessible to users with visual impairments. In *Proceedings of the 12th international ACM SIGACCESS conference on computers and accessibility* (pp. 187–194). https://doi.org/10.1145/1878803.1878837

Little, L. M., Dean, E., Tomchek, S., & Dunn, W. (2017). Sensory processing patterns in autism, attention deficit hyperactivity disorder, and typical development. *Physical & Occupational Therapy In Pediatrics*, 1–12. https://doi.org/10.1080/01942638.2017.1390809

Liu, T., Thiebaut de Schotten, M., Altarelli, I., Ramus, F., & Zhao, J. (2022). Neural dissociation of visual attention span and phonological deficits in developmental dyslexia: A hub-based white matter network analysis. *Human Brain Mapping, 43*(17), 5210–5219. https://doi.org/10.1002/hbm.25997

Lopes, P., Ion, A., Mueller, W., Hoffmann, D., Jonell, P., & Baudisch, P. (2015). Proprioceptive interaction. In *Proceedings of the 33rd annual ACM conference on human factors in computing systems* (pp. 939–948). https://doi.org/10.1145/2702123.2702461

Mikkelsen, M., Wodka, E. L., Mostofsky, S. H., & Puts, N. A. J. (2018). Autism spectrum disorder in the scope of tactile processing. *Developmental Cognitive Neuroscience, 29*, 140–150. https://doi.org/10.1016/j.dcn.2016.12.005

Monica, I., Cibrian, F. L., Chavez, E., & Tentori, M. (2023a). Using a small dataset to classify strength-interactions with an elastic display: A case study for the screening of autism spectrum disorder. *International Journal of Machine Learning and Cybernetics, 14*(1), 151–169. https://doi.org/10.1007/s13042-022-01554-2

Monica, I., Tentori, M., & Cibrian, F. L. (2023b). Understanding the musical interaction of children with autism spectrum disorder using elastic display. *Personal and Ubiquitous Computing*. https://doi.org/10.1007/s00779-022-01703-y

Mottron, L., Dawson, M., Soulières, I., Hubert, B., & Burack, J. (2006). Enhanced perceptual functioning in autism: An update, and eight principles of autistic perception. *Journal of Autism and Developmental Disorders, 36*(1), 27–43. https://doi.org/10.1007/s10803-005-0040-7

Myles, B. S. (2001). Understanding the hidden curriculum: An essential social skill for children and youth with asperger syndrome. *Intervention in School and Clinic, 36*(5), 279–286. https://doi.org/10.1177/105345120103600504

Oh, U., & Findlater, L. (2015). A performance comparison of on-hand versus on-phone nonvisual input by blind and sighted users. *ACM Transactions on Accessible Computing, 7*(4), 14:1–14:20. https://doi.org/10.1145/2820616

Parsons, S. (2000). Development of social skills amongst adults with Asperger's Syndrome using virtual environments. *Virtual Reality*.

Parsons, S., & Cobb, S. (2011). State-of-the-art of virtual reality technologies for children on the autism spectrum. *European Journal of Special Needs Education, 26*(3), 355–366. https://doi.org/10.1080/08856257.2011.593831

Parsons, S., Leonard, A., & Mitchell, P. (2006). Virtual environments for social skills training: Comments from two adolescents with autistic spectrum disorder. *Computers & Education, 47*(2), 186–206. https://doi.org/10.1016/j.compedu.2004.10.003

Piper, A. M., O'Brien, E., Morris, M. R., & Winograd, T. (2006). SIDES: A cooperative tabletop computer game for social skills development. In *Proceedings of the 2006 20th anniversary conference on computer supported cooperative work* (pp. 1–10). https://doi.org/10.1145/1180875.1180877

Ratanasit, D., & Moore, M. M. (2005). Representing graphical user interfaces with sound: A review of approaches. *Journal of Visual Impairment & Blindness, 99*(2), 69–84. https://doi.org/10.1177/0145482X0509900202

Reid, L. G., & Snow-Weaver, A. (2008). WCAG 2.0: A web accessibility standard for the evolving web. In *Proceedings of the 2008 international cross-disciplinary conference on web accessibility (W4A)* (pp. 109–115). https://doi.org/10.1145/1368044.1368069

Rello, L., & Baeza-Yates, R. (2016). The effect of font type on screen readability by people with dyslexia. *ACM Transactions on Accessible Computing, 8*(4), 1–33. https://doi.org/10.1145/2897736

Rello, L., & Bigham, J. P. (2017). Good background colors for readers: A study of people with and without dyslexia. In *Proceedings of the 19th international ACM SIGACCESS conference on computers and accessibility* (pp. 72–80). https://doi.org/10.1145/3132525.3132546

Ringland, K. E., Wolf, C. T., Boyd, L., Brown, J. K., Palermo, A., Lakes, K., & Hayes, G. R. (2019). DanceCraft: A whole-body interactive system for children with autism. In *Proceedings of the 21st international ACM SIGACCESS conference on computers and accessibility* (pp. 572–574). https://doi.org/10.1145/3308561.3354604

Ringland, K. E., Zalapa, R., Neal, M., Escobedo, L., Tentori, M. E., & Hayes, G. R. (2014). SensoryPaint: A natural user interface supporting sensory integration in children with neurodevelopmental disorders. In *Proceedings of the extended abstracts of the 32nd annual ACM conference on human factors in computing systems* (pp. 1681–1686). https://doi.org/10.1145/2559206.2581249

Robertson, C. E., & Baron-Cohen, S. (2017). Sensory perception in autism. *Nature Reviews Neuroscience, 18*(11), 671–684. https://doi.org/10.1038/nrn.2017.112

Röder, B., Rösler, F., & Neville, H. J. (2001). Auditory memory in congenitally blind adults: A behavioral-electrophysiological investigation. *Cognitive Brain Research, 11*(2), 289–303. https://doi.org/10.1016/S0926-6410(01)00002-7

Roley, S. S., Mailloux, Z., Parham, L. D., Schaaf, R. C., Lane, C. J., & Cermak, S. (2014). Sensory integration and praxis patterns in children with autism. *American Journal of Occupational Therapy, 69*(1), 6901220010p1. https://doi.org/10.5014/ajot.2015.012476

Schauder, K. B., Mash, L. E., Bryant, L. K., & Cascio, C. J. (2015). Interoceptive ability and body awareness in autism spectrum disorder. *Journal of Experimental Child Psychology, 131*, 193–200

Schulze, M., Aslan, B., Stöcker, T., Stirnberg, R., Lux, S., & Philipsen, A. (2021). Disentangling early versus late audiovisual integration in adult ADHD: A combined behavioural and resting-state connectivity study. *Journal of Psychiatry and Neuroscience, 46*(5), E528–E537. https://doi.org/10.1503/jpn.210017

Schulze, M., Lux, S., & Philipsen, A. (2020). *Sensory processing in adult ADHD—A systematic review* [Preprint]. In Review. https://doi.org/10.21203/rs.3.rs-71514/v1

Sean, V. (2020). *Connecting the dots for people with autism: A data-driven approach to designing and evaluating a global filter* [Ph.D., Chapman University]. https://www.proquest.com/docview/2405147159/abstract/234B7B9218144E8EPQ/1

Selinger, C. (n.d.). Auditory processing or listening comprehension? *Brooklyn Letters*. Retrieved March 15, 2023, from https://brooklynletters.com/whats-the-difference-between-auditory-processing-and-listening-comprehension/

Shah, P. (2016). Interoception: The Eighth Sensory System: Practical Solutions for Improving Self-Regulation, Self-Awareness and Social Understanding of Individuals with Autism Spectrum and Related Disorders: KJ Mahler: Shawnee Mission KS, AAPC, 2015, 186 pp, $29.95 (paper), ISBN 978-1-942197-14-0

Simm, W., Ferrario, M. A., Gradinar, A., & Whittle, J. (2014). Prototyping "clasp": Implications for designing digital technology for and with adults with autism. In *Proceedings of the 2014 conference on designing interactive systems* (pp. 345–354). https://doi.org/10.1145/2598510.260 0880

Sonuga-Barke, E. J. S., & Fairchild, G. (2012). Neuroeconomics of attention-deficit/hyperactivity disorder: Differential influences of medial, dorsal, and ventral prefrontal brain networks on suboptimal decision making? *Biological Psychiatry, 72*(2), 126–133. https://doi.org/10.1016/j.bio psych.2012.04.004

Tactile Processing, Part 1. (n.d.). Perkins school for the blind. Retrieved March 15, 2023, from https://www.perkins.org/resource/tactile-processing-part-1/

Takahashi, I., Oki, M., Bourreau, B., Kitahara, I., & Suzuki, K. (2018). FUTUREGYM: A gymnasium with interactive floor projection for children with special needs. *International Journal of Child-Computer Interaction, 15*, 37–47. https://doi.org/10.1016/j.ijcci.2017.12.002

Tavassoli, T., Bellesheim, K., Tommerdahl, M., Holden, J. M., Kolevzon, A., & Buxbaum, J. D. (2016). Altered tactile processing in children with autism spectrum disorder. *Autism Research, 9*(6), 616–620. https://doi.org/10.1002/aur.1563

Viirre, E., Lorant, Z., Draper, M., & Furness III, T. A. (2001). Virtual reality and the vestibular system: a brief review. *Information Technologies in Medicine: Rehabilitation and Treatment, 2*, 101–108

Williams, Z. J., Suzman, E., Bordman, S. L., Markfeld, J. E., Kaiser, S. M., Dunham, K. A., Zoltowski, A. R., Failla, M. D., Cascio, C. J., & Woynaroski, T. G. (2023). Characterizing interoceptive differences in autism: A systematic review and meta-analysis of case–control studies. *Journal of Autism and Developmental Disorders, 53*(3), 947–962. https://doi.org/10.1007/s10803-022-05656-2

Yaneva, V., Temnikova, I., & Mitkov, R. (2015). Accessible texts for autism: An eye-tracking study. In *Proceedings of the 17th international ACM SIGACCESS conference on computers & accessibility—ASSETS '15* (pp. 49–57). https://doi.org/10.1145/2700648.2809852

Yu, W., & Brewster, S. (2003). Evaluation of multimodal graphs for blind people. *Universal Access in the Information Society, 2*(2), 105–124. https://doi.org/10.1007/s10209-002-0042-6

Designing Sensory Environments and Sensory Interactions in Virtual Reality

4

Autism and Sensory Perception

Humans continually integrate multiple sensory modalities to understand the world around them. Individual sensory modalities can be challenging to process for people with autism, but a particular challenge is multi modal integration. Because of the complex sensory experience, many autistic people may prefer lean information, such as text messaging or use a single channel–unisensory—such as writing emails (Howard & Sedgewick, 2021). Some researchers have leveraged a preference for lean media to support communication practice using an expressionless robot (Daniel, 2017).

Specific challenges exist in autism regarding integrating visuo-spatial, auditory-temporal, global–local processing). These challenges occur to the degree that researchers hypothesize that autistic people may engage in *channel switching*. For example, they may use "visual processing, versus auditory, as a strategy to engage with the environments" and they may also use *sensory conservation* by reducing visual input which in turn reduces auditory sensory load to conserve senses (Lachmann et al., 2014; Little et al., 2017). As a note, there are several superior perceptual abilities that exist among some people with autism (Mottron et al., 2006). It is important to note that these strengths can be leveraged to improve delivering information in assistive technology systems. This Chapter explores ways to leverage strengths and work around weaknesses, and considers the design of multiple sensory profiles (Dunn, 2014) as user requirements in the same system. First by incorporating Dunn's neurological threshold continuum (Dunn, 2014) as user require-ments of the computing environments, then consider the self-regulation continuum as user requirements for interaction design (Dunn, 2014).

L. Boyd, *The Sensory Accommodation Framework for Technology*, Synthesis Lectures on Technology and Health, https://doi.org/10.1007/978-3-031-48843-6_4

In Occupational Therapy clinics, a survey, The He Sensory Profile 2™ (Dunn, 2014)[1] for children ages 3 to 14:11 years old, provides explanation of the survey results of the caregiver survey (Dunn, 2014). The survey asks caregivers to rate on likert scale: almost always (90% or more of the time), frequently (75% of the time), half the time (50% of the time), occasionally (25% of the time), almost never (10% or less of the time) or does not apply (unable to answer because this behavior has not been observed or does not apply) across the sensory processing domains of auditory, visual, touch, movement, body position, and oral. Additional domains include conduct, social emotional and attentional responses associated with sensory processing. These domains are distributed across four factors: seekers, avoiders, sensors, and bystanders. These quadrants of Dunn's Sensory processing framework are divided by the axes of self-regulation continuum that spans from passive to active and the neurological threshold continuum that spans from low to high (Dunn, 2014).

The Sensory Profile 2™ (Dunn, 2014) provides intersecting axes to group profiles into quadrants. These axes can be aligned with interaction design goals by considering passive to active self-regulation in terms of the user's interactions with the system and the low to high neurological thresholds as the intensity of sensory features in the virtual environment and customizing user control to support the continuum of self-regulation behavior–see Chap. 4 for details. Applying Dunn's Sensory Processing framework to interaction design along with user's preferences to technology allows us to blend stakeholder's needs through customized and comfortable software for neurodiverse users, see Chap. 5 for full details.

Sensory Environment as Support the Neurological Threshold Continuum

The Sensory Profile 2™ User manual (Dunn, 2014) describes the neurological threshold the central nervous system has as a limit of how much stimulation can be processed. If someone has a low neurological threshold, they will be responsive very quickly or with small amounts of stimulation where someone with a high threshold would require more or longer stimulation to reach a place where they can process information. The neurological threshold is the balance point where the person is receiving enough information to be aware and attentive, but not too much to be overwhelmed (Dunn, 2014). In other words, someone with a low neurological threshold may be seen as overly sensitive to stimulation where someone with a high neurological threshold might seem under sensitive or hyposensitive to stimulation.

The Sensory-Environment can be designed for a continuum of neurological thresholds. This would expand the accessibility to divergent users; however, the requirements

---

[1] The Sensory Profile 2™ Assessment can be purchased by clinicians at https://www.pearsonasses sments.com/store/usassessments/en/Store/Professional-Assessments/Motor-Sensory/Sensory-Pro file-2/p/100000822.html.

can contradict one another as points along the axis become further apart. For example, at the high threshold end of the axis, users are believed to be habituating to sensory input (Little et al., 2017) and may require additional inputs to regulate their engagement; whereas at the low threshold end, users remain sensitive (Dunn, 2014) and may become overwhelmed with low levels of sensory input over time. A person's sensory processing needs as well as the characteristics of a task (e.g., does the task require integrating multiple modalities continually over time?) should be part of the system requirements of an assistive technology. Because all information from the physical world gets paired down to by the technologist, there is potential to leave out information that allows for customizing the information for a holistic view or the detailed view (e.g., map view or list of written directions). The ability to switch between views such as a map of an area or verbal instructions is now common, however both views may still not meet a neurodiverse users' sensory processing needs.

Sensory Interaction as Support for Self-Regulation

The Sensory Profile 2™ User manual describes the Behavioral Response axis as "The way people behave to manage their own needs. At one end of this continuum, children respond passively in relation to their thresholds. This means that they have a tendency to let things happen and then respond. At the other end of the behavioral continuum, children respond actively in relation to their thresholds this means they work to control the amount and type of sensory input they receive" (Dunn, 2014). When a person or caregiver for someone completes the detailed survey about all the sensory systems and their sensory experiences, the results provide areas that are needed for typical, hypo or hyper-reactive. These become goals for occupational therapists to address in therapy, however, technical systems must also utilize these user's needs in systems to ensure systems are accessible to people with very diverse sensory experiences.

Designing Virtual Environments for All 4 Sensory Quadrants

To integrate the concepts from the Sensory Profile 2™ user information was collected from The Sensory Profile 2™ manual for children ages 3 to 14:11 years old. The manual that provides explanation for the survey results of the caregiver survey (Dunn, 2014). The survey asks caregivers to rate several items on Likert scale: almost always (90% or more of the time), frequently (75% of the time), half the time (50% of the time), occasionally (25% of the time), almost never (10% or less of the time) or does not apply (unable to answer because this behavior has not been observed or does not apply) across the sensory processing domains of auditory, visual, touch, movement, body position, and oral. Additional domains include conduct, social, emotional, and attentional responses associated with sensory processing. These domains are distributed across four possible factors: seekers, avoiders, sensors, and bystanders. Results of The Sensory Profile 2™ (Dunn, 2014) reveal that quadrants represent the interaction between the thresholds to stimulation axis and the passive to active engagement with the environment. The quadrants provide four distinct profiles that Dunn calls Bystander: degree child misses sensory input Seeker: degree child obtains sensory input; Avoider: degree child is bothered by sensory input; Sensor: degree child detects sensory input (Dunn, 2014).

Case Study for Sensory Diversity in Multiplayer VR Apps

vrSensory is a suite of games designed to meet a wide range of sensory profiles so that children can play comfortably and together regardless of their sensory preferences or needs. Employing a user centered approach to design and evaluation, vrSensory (Boyd, 2018; Boyd et al., 2019), resulted in five custom virtual reality applications. Each was designed based primarily around one of the four distinct sensory patterns that categorize the continuum of human sensory experience in The Sensory Profile 2™ (Dunn, 2014). Additionally, a fifth application was built for the "typical sensory processing" style.

Case Study Participants

The three diverse children displayed bystander, seeker, and typical patterns. These terms will also be referred to as *sensory personas*. Addressing each person's preferences as well as whole also addressing his diversity of preferences became the primary system requirements for a virtual space that would be comfortable for each child to play in alone and together. Each of the three children picked a theme for their desired virtual environments. The bystander child picked watching thunderstorms, the seeker child picked an area to sing and dance in as the star, and the typical sensory profile child picked his favorite pastime–playing baseball. After each participant chose the type of activity they wanted to engage in, then the interactions for each environment were designed to meet needs and wants for 3 participants according to their profiles. The child's chosen activity and their sensory persona were the primary factors in the design, it is noteworthy that they are neurodiverse in that the bystander has autism and motor difficulties, the seeker has ADHD, and the third child score was reported as typically developing (Table 4.1).

Bystander's Choice: Thunderstorm

In Thunderstorm, the users are spawned into a desert scene, where they stand and can see hills, a few trees, and rain coming down. There is thunder and rain audio, as well as bolts and flashes of lightning. When a lightning flash occurs, the sky) lights up with a colorful, cloud-filled storm. A player can walk around or teleport and if others are in the system,

Table 4.1 Main interaction design by each sensory persona for each VR application

Sensory environment	Bystander[1] interactions	Seeker[2] interactions	Avoider[3] interactions	Sensor[4] interactions
Thunderstorm[1]	Passive interaction (watching high intensity thunderstorm)	User agency to create endless, rapid movement around planet via teleporting	Can move to hide inside mountains	Can turn off volume, dim screen for less intensity
Dance[2]	Has automated multiple input sources for audio and video	Has three larger than life screens of constraint input to switch between, can dance, sing, choose song	Can view the screen of choosing to dance or sing or avoiding. No enforcement or feedback from the system is provided	Can coordinate dance moves and singing through continuous video feed
Laser tag[3]	Can stay behind protective barriers and shoot at robots	Can be running and dodging and shooting throughout the maze	Can be in a high action area while behind a protective barrier	Can hide, stay still, and predict when they might need to move
Horseback riding[4]	Can let horse lead though nature on predetermined path	Can speed up or slow down the horse, take the horse off path, into lakes, underwater	Can watch the horse or others on horses walk through the scene	User can sit while horse walks guided path through mountains countryside
Baseball[5]	Can widen target range of bat to increase hits	Can swing as hard as they like and send ball out of the park	Can observe from the stands	Can remain stationary with small movements resulting in big hits

[1]Intermittent loud noise and high contrast lights,
[2]Multiple jumbotrons with 3 different types of audio—visual stimulation synced to a song
[3]Maze as a playing field with barriers to hide behind as robots ascend on the field in a predictable pattern
[4]User stands or sits on chair or today while horse takes a walk-through nature
[5]User stands or sits to swing a physical bat to hit a virtual baseball

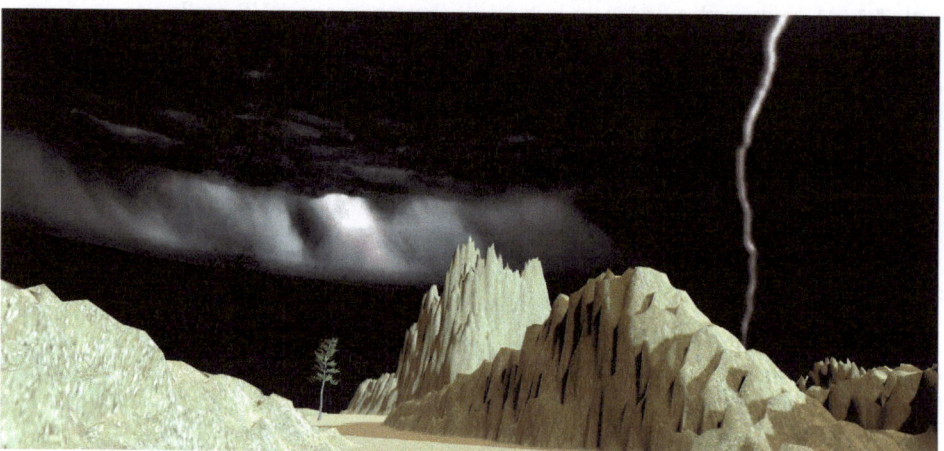

Fig. 4.1 Screenshot of the thunderstorm application that was designed primarily for a bystander profile. The fast flash of movement and contrast in luminance between the bright lightning and the dark sky is intended to provide intense stimulation for the high neurological threshold. With regard to the self-regulation continuum, the thundersorm module is a passive one where no action need be taken, the user can simply enjoy the visual display of thunder and rain

they can chat. This is designed to be a somewhat passive interaction with high intensity stimulation (Fig. 4.1).

The thunderstorm app was designed for the bystander as his preferred activity. Given that other profiles would be included in the virtual play, the system was designed also for seeker and for as well as for an avoider persona in anticipation that other children might join in the future.

Seeker's Choice: Dance and Sing

Dance

The Dance Arena in Sensory is a stage set with three jumbotron screens each with a different aspect of auditory and or visual stimulation that is synchronized to a pop song of the user's choice. The song is playing with the lyrics showing on one screen, a music video is shown on the middle screen and an avatar showing dance moves is shown on the third screen the user is spawned into the center of the stage and can move around, and initiate their own dance moves can coordinate with a partner orient toward an audience (Boyd, 2019). Sensor (Horseback Riding) (Fig. 4.2).

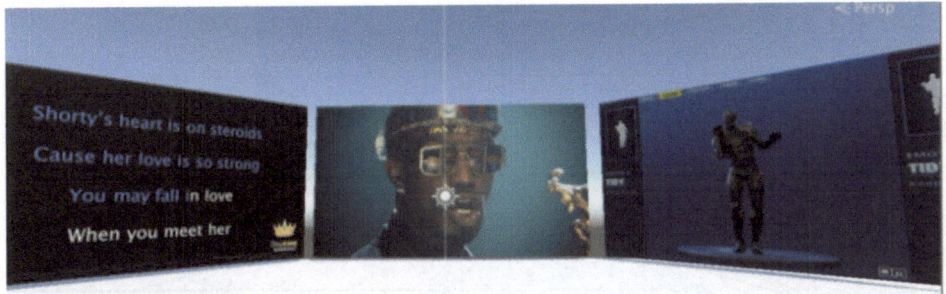

Fig. 4.2 Screenshot of three screens on the stage for Dance and Sing Application designed primarily for a Seeker profile. To address the high neurological threshold, there is an abundance of stimulation occurring at High intensities, large-scale jumbotrons which are synchronized to provide the music video, sing-along lyrics and dance-along moves to the song of the user's choice. In relation to the self-regulation continuum, the large space is open for movement and dance as well as for others to join in

Horseback Riding

In Horseback Riding, the user is spawned onto a horse (and in the physical world they sit on a yoga ball or chair) and can bounce along with the horse if they choose. The horse animation depicts the horse's head bobbing up and down in their foreground as it walks on a predetermined path unless the user pushes a button on the remote control to set off on a new path. This design affords very pleasant passive interaction with a low level of stimulation as the virtual world rendered in low ploy to reduce detail. Additionally, a user can use controls to speed up the horse pace (Fig. 4.3).

Avoider (Laser Tag)

Laser Tag

The laser tag game takes place in a maze and is designed primarily for the avoider profile, barriers are placed on the playing field for the user to be in the action but protected by the shelter. Robots patrol the playing field and shoot lasers at users. The robots are spawned into predictable locations and the user may also choose to shoot back at the robots. This game provides low levels of environmental stimulation and is highly active about maintaining a low level of stimulation (Boyd, 2019) (Fig. 4.4).

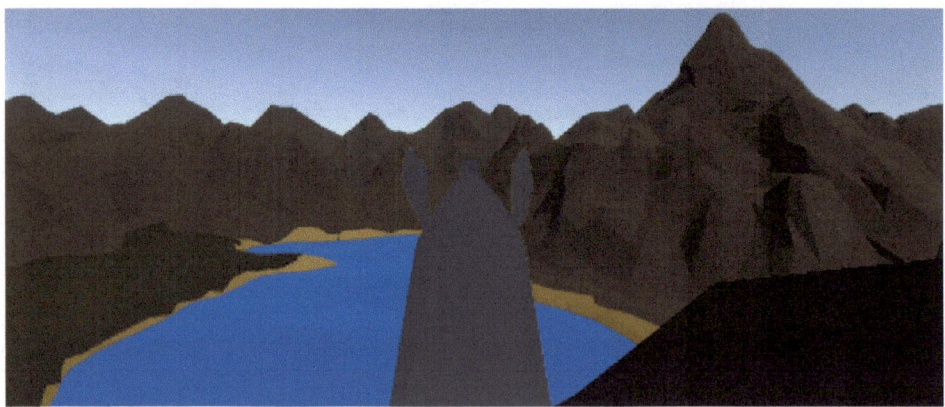

Fig. 4.3 Screenshot from horseback of walk through the mountains was primarily designed for the sensor profile to contain a low poly environment to not be overly detailed and distracting visually and low user interaction where the user simply can sit on the horse as it walks through the countryside

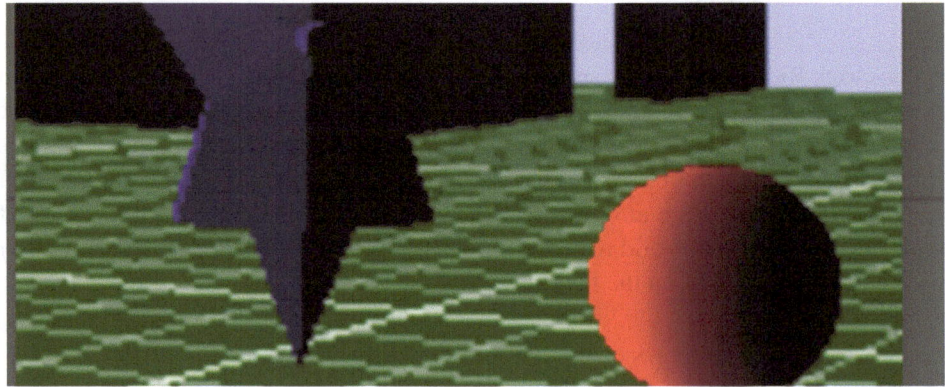

Fig. 4.4 Screenshot of the laser tag application which was primarily developed for the avoider profile. Given this profile has a low threshold dissimulation, the environment is very simple, and the user interactions though are designed for a physically active user who can dodge robots who shoot at them, as well as run around barriers to shoot back at the robots

Typical (Baseball)

Baseball

In the baseball system, the batter spawns into the system at the batter's box and is holding a physical baseball bat. When the ball is pitched, the batter can swing to hit the ball and can see the ball flying through the stadium. This role is intended to be moderately active with moderate stimulation (Boyd, 2019) (Fig. 4.5).

The Role of Movement in Interaction Design

In close association with sensory perception is the ability to move (see Fig. 4.6 where sensory perception and motor processing occur in the same ring). Being able to move one's body through space is essential to a sense of agency, autonomy, and independence. Children with motor disabilities/challenges are an underserved community as the work to rehabilitate the body and mind is extensive. This work not only involves the child working toward therapy goals but also family members, therapists, teachers, and caregivers providing support to engage in activities of daily living. To improve physical therapy outcomes related to ambulation and navigation, practice outside of therapy is required. Physical therapists may recommend practicing activities of daily living outside the clinic when a child is ready, however, they are often met with resistance. This type of practice is often a challenge for caregivers who do not feel equipped to provide the level of assistance required; fear the child may get hurt; or are otherwise not able to support practicing the motor skills needed to improve independence.

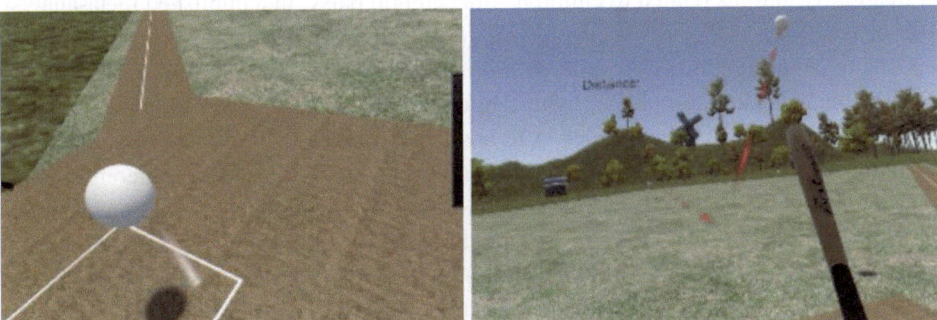

Fig. 4.5 Screenshot of two views in the Baseball application. Left is the baseball coming toward the batter. Right is the ball flying out to the outfield with a virtual view of the bat. The baseball app was designed for a typical he Sensory Profile 2™. The user interacts by swinging a physical bat which is represented digitally in the virtual environment

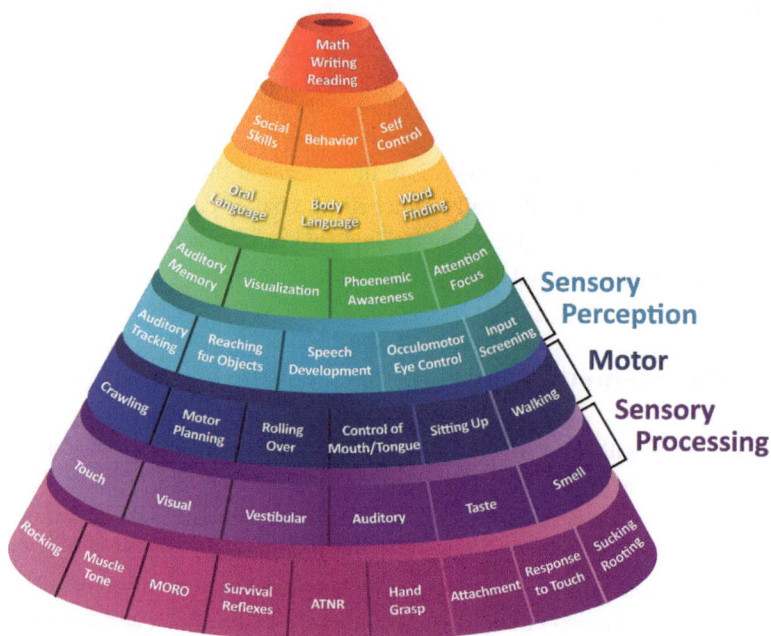

Fig. 4.6 Learning skills pyramid showing motor skills a layer between sensory perception and sensory processing skills

Case Study in Movement Therapy

VR as a playful way to motivate children with Cerebral Palsy to participate in leisure activities and therapy activities is not a new idea. Virtual reality is an emerging modality for treating symptoms related to children with cerebral palsy. In a published meta-analysis, 70% of reviewed works revealed positive results in brain reorganization, motor skills, or visual spatial outcomes for children with cerebral palsy (Bryanton et al., 2006). The authors conclude that compliance with therapy would be high given the motivating and engaging aspects that VR provides. VR has been found to be motivating and feasible Bryanton et al., 2006) as parents and children both reported positive outcomes. "Even the youngest children were able to complete the tasks within the virtual environments and generate movements necessary to interact with the virtual objects" (Bryanton et al., 2006). However, as an emerging field, little has been explored regarding benefits beyond the research or clinic. Traditional therapy attempts provide opportunities to create new motor patterns and then transfer the newly acquired motor pattern from the training site to activities of daily living. Transfer of skill has been observed through VR-based balance intervention with traumatic brain injury patients as well as children with cerebral palsy (Bryanton et al., 2006).

Virtual reality has been an important addition to therapy that researchers have measured the playfulness of children in the system. Test of Playfulness was used to measure play with children with Cerebral Palsy in virtual reality systems. The authors found that "environments which allowed creativity, expression, and control over the activity were the most motivating. Environments that did not have good timing and reaction time to user inputs were frustrating. Environments should not be too challenging so that the skills of the user are not matched to the requirements of the program and this is frustrating" (Reid, 2004). Along with a physical therapist, parent, and child with autism and cerebral palsy, I explored vrSensory as immersive virtual play spaces bridge the gap in between physical therapists' recommendations and parents' confidence that a child is ready and able to take the next steps in rehabilitation at home. Over the course of multiple phases, this work will explore sensory-comfortable spaces that encourage movement.

The child participant's survey revealed he is *missing sensory information more than others*—as reflected by a high score on the neurological threshold continuum and low score on the self-regulation continuum, this child scored in the Sensor as described in (Dunn, 2014). Because vrSensory was already designed for easy entry, a child participant was invited to come into play in the sensory-inclusive modules. He was accompanied by his father, grandmother, and physical therapist. He was fearful of putting on the headset for the first 30 min. During this warmup time, his physical therapist and father took turns wearing the headset with him standing or sitting nearby with the physical bat that was also represented in the virtual game. The child participant could see the virtual world on a laptop, so it was moved to be in his sight of view. The child participant, his father and Physical Therapist playfully explored this dynamic for a while allowing the child participant time to get comfortable with the headset. Over time, the child participant put the headset on his father and PT, and then his father invited him to put it on. Once he put the headset on, he took a moment to explore the 3D environment. He looked down at his shadow on the ground and the cartoon hand that accompanied his avatar. He spoke about these elements. Since he showed interest in exploring 3D environments, he was invited to try the other two applications available on the server. He adeptly noticed the conference poster on the wall where the screenshots of the modules were displayed and started talking about them. He entered the thunderstorm application where he looked up at the rain. He did not walk around and the remote was not working properly to show him how to teleport so he was invited to try horseback riding. He vigorously bounced on the yoga ball with his physical therapist helping, giggling along the way.

The child participant's father commented that having the modules displayed on a large screen at the start could help children understand the VR system quickly, and that the freedom to explore the room and the virtual environment was a big reason he was so motivated to play. This engaging space provided a shared context for his Physical Therapist to provide physical support and to comment on and play along such as making horse noises and other sound effects.

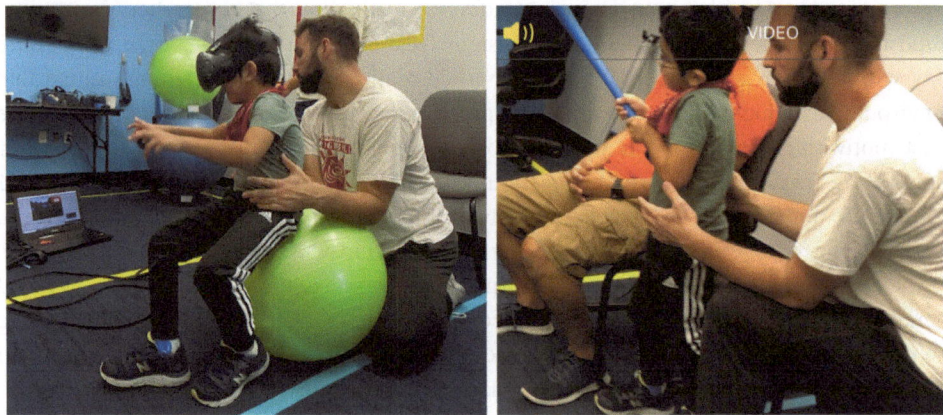

Fig. 4.7 Sensor participant on yoga ball in horseback riding application with support to his core from his physical therapist

vrSensory was used in work to motivate repetitive motor skill routine as seen in Fig. 4.7 where a child participant with cerebral palsy and autism, physically, is now comfortable being in VR. His motivation has increased for engaging in repetitive physical therapy movements that occurred several times a week because now they're applied to a leisure activity like swinging about at a virtual baseball. This platform made that activity also accessible for him as he required support to swing a bat.

Using the motor practice goal as an example of sensory-environment first design allowed the child work toward moving independently is now an actionable goal as he's getting the repetition, he needs to support the mixed reality environment. Lastly, how learnable is the system for the user? With ongoing practice, the student is able to learn the skill because he has the tangible objects, the motivation, the physical support, the comfort of being in VR, and the motivation is understandable to him. He's able to effectively engage with the system and his therapist. These goals allow for guardrails to be in place to ensure everyone can be satisfied with innovations.

Implication for Design of the Sensory Environment Layer

Figure 4.8 illustrates the sensory environment layer of the sensory accommodation framework. In viewing this layer one can see that as sensory input travels into the learning cone from the bottom up by the time it reaches the sensory layer multiple mechanisms can support processing. On the left there is a 8-point star letting in a large amount of sensory input and the strategy would be a smaller star to filter out some of it in other words reducing the amount of that kind of and put that's being received by the hypersensitive neurological threshold of the user. In the middle there's a moon shape showing that not all the signal is being received. This would be for someone who is hypersensitive, the circle augmentation fills out the missing piece of information by adding to what is understood by the user.

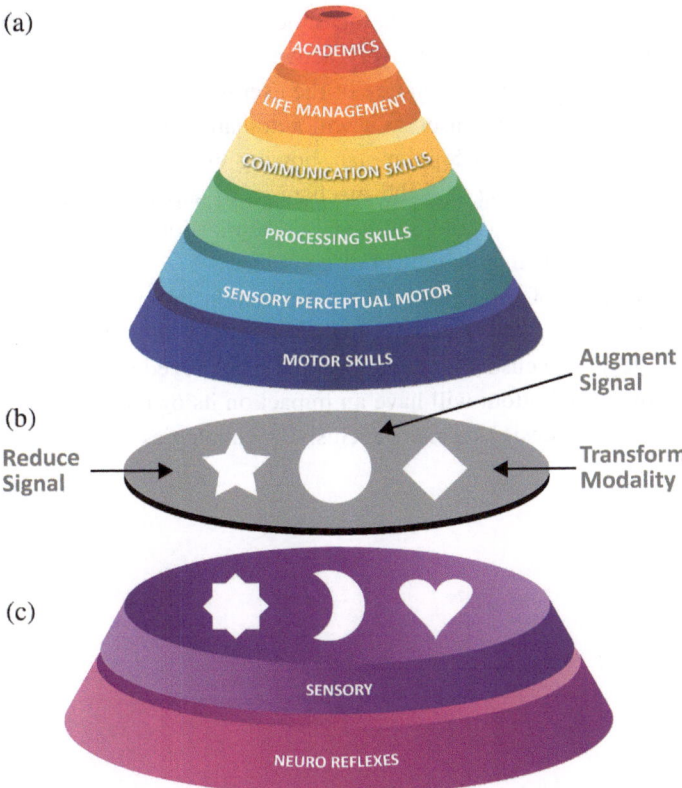

Fig. 4.8 Sensory environment layer of the sensory accommodation framework. Three mechanisms were derived for the purpose of designing systems: **a** Channel reduction: removing information from the environment, **b** Channel augmentation: adding information to the environment, **c** Channel transformation: changing the form of information

The heart-shaped opening in the learning cone allows in a specific modality that may not be well interpreted so the mechanism here is to change the modality to transform it into a different input type, so for example if it is auditory information to transform it into visual information.

Implication for Design Sensory Interaction Layer

The sensory interaction layer represents opportunities at the motor level of the learning cone (Fig. 4.9). As sensory input begins at the bottom and is funneled up toward the top, this is a stage when motor actions are processed and an opportunity to design mechanisms to support a range of self-regulation behaviors. Figure 4.7 presents design opportunities at the sensory perceptual motor level of the learning cone. The mechanisms to support sensory interactions are presented at two ends of a spectrum; one is to fully automate user interaction for a passive self-regulation style and the other is to highly customize as much interaction as possible for the very active self-regulation style. On the left, is a square that is the absence or passive nature of the user to change their environment, in the filter layer it's automated for the user so it will automatically happen as indicated by the filled in square on the right is a 5-point star showing the average amount of interaction that may be available to a user and the mechanism to support someone with a highly active self-regulation style is to add additional customization features so the eight-point star indicates more options than is typical of a system.

The recommendation of the Sensory Accommodation Framework is to start building from the bottom and play all the strategies that relate to that ring of development and then move to the next level and ensure those strategies are employed as well as the information that is adjusted from the bottom will have an impact on its own through the process there are additional places for designing more inclusive technologies.

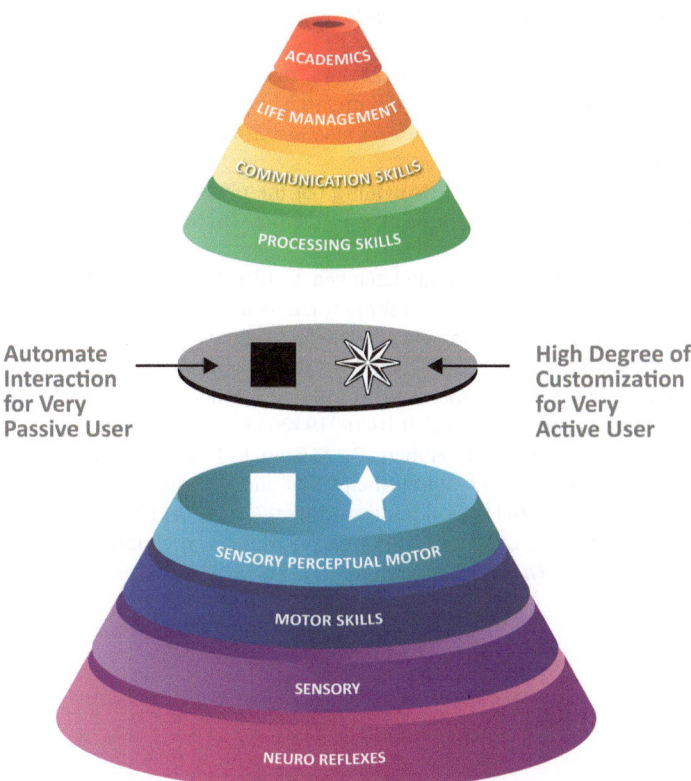

Fig. 4.9 Sensory interaction layer of the sensory accommodation framework. Left is the mechanism to automate an interaction for a passive user and to the right is a mechanism to highly customize user interaction for an active user in relation to one's self-regulation behavior

References

Boyd, L. (2019). Designing sensory-inclusive virtual play spaces for children. In *Proceedings of the 18th ACM international conference on interaction design and children* (pp. 446–451). https://doi.org/10.1145/3311927.3325315

Boyd, L. E. (2018). *Designing and evaluating alternative channels: Visualizing nonverbal communication through AR and VR systems for people with autism.* https://escholarship.org/content/qt04t4f3v6/qt04t4f3v6.pdf

Boyd, L., Day, K., Abdo, K., Wasserman, B., Hayes, G., & Linstead, E. (2019, May). Paper prototyping comfortable VR play for diverse sensory needs. In *Proceedings of ACM CHI conference on human factors in computing systems (CHI'19).* https://doi.org/10.1145/10.1145/3290607.3313080

Bryanton, C., Bossé, J., Brien, M., Mclean, J., McCormick, A., & Sveistrup, H. (2006). Feasibility, motivation, and selective motor control: Virtual reality compared to conventional home exercise in children with cerebral palsy. *CyberPsychology & Behavior, 9*(2), 123–128. https://doi.org/10.1089/cpb.2006.9.123

Daniel, J. (2017). Use of lean robotic communication to improve social response of children with autism. *SSRN Electronic Journal.* https://doi.org/10.2139/ssrn.3733701

Dunn, W. (2014). *He sensory profile 2™ user's manual: Strengths-based approach to assessment and planning.* Pearson.

Howard, P. L., & Sedgewick, F. (2021). 'Anything but the phone!': Communication mode preferences in the autism community. *Autism, 25*(8), 2265–2278. https://doi.org/10.1177/13623613211014995

Lachmann, T., Schmitt, A., Braet, W., & van Leeuwen, C. (2014). Letters in the forest: Global precedence effect disappears for letters but not for non-letters under reading-like conditions. *Frontiers in Psychology, 5.* https://www.frontiersin.org/articles/10.3389/fpsyg.2014.00705

Little, L. M., Dean, E., Tomchek, S., & Dunn, W. (2017). sensory processing patterns in autism, attention deficit hyperactivity disorder, and typical development. *Physical & Occupational Therapy in Pediatrics*, 1–12.https://doi.org/10.1080/01942638.2017.1390809

Mottron, L., Dawson, M., Soulières, I., Hubert, B., & Burack, J. (2006). Enhanced perceptual functioning in autism: An update, and eight principles of autistic perception. *Journal of Autism and Developmental Disorders, 36*(1), 27–43. https://doi.org/10.1007/s10803-005-0040-7

Reid, D. (2004). The influence of virtual reality on playfulness in children with cerebral palsy: A pilot study. *Occupational Therapy International, 11*(3), 131–144. https://doi.org/10.1002/oti.202

The Hierarchy of Visual Attention in Natural Scenes

5

Part 1: The Hidden Hierarchy of Global and Local Visual Processing

Visual attention has been a major focus of cognitive research related to autism for the past 60 years (Abdo & Al Osman, 2019; Almourad & Bataineh, 2020; Amso et al., 2014; Baisa et al., 2021; Bertone et al., 2005; Brooks et al., 1968; de Jong et al., 2008; Deruelle et al., 2004; Gargaro et al., 2018; Grinter et al., 2010; Gross, 2005; Guy et al., 2016; Hayward et al., 2018; Hill et al., 2014; Koh et al., 2010; Lovaas et al., 1979; Rinehart et al., 2000a; Robertson & Baron-Cohen, 2017; Townsend et al., 1996; Wang et al., 2007). Many theories exist about the neurological underpinnings of autistic visual attention as well as holistic accounts from autistic scholars—monotropism—the propensity to have a singular focus—as a defining feature of autism. Visual attention occurs at the preconscious and conscious phases, and therefore offers a unique opportunity to bridge these separate processing workflows. Processing is rapid and it occurs in an ongoing fashion as what to attend to in the physical world is persistently around us and in movement. Filtering visual content depends on context and needs and the human state. The fields of neuroergonomics and neuroeconomics discuss how our brains make trade-offs regarding information and how these can be translated into technologies. This chapter provides a deep dive into visual attention and specifically in autism and then into ways to augment automatic processes to offload some of the burden of filtering out irrelevant information.

Visual attention is a complex concept that requires an understanding of the integration of low-level sensory processing and high-level cognition processing. Each of these streams of information has a unique role in visual attention. Two of these levels (global and local) are often differentiated by where they fall in terms of the human information

L. Boyd, *The Sensory Accommodation Framework for Technology*, Synthesis Lectures on Technology and Health, https://doi.org/10.1007/978-3-031-48843-6_5

processing workflow with low-level being the initial input much like the stack in the computer architecture with the low level taking in sensory input from the world and compiling it into information that is fed forward to the global, higher-level processors and becoming conscious.

Hierarchical Dimension of Visual Attention

One theory that has strong evidence in the clinical fields but very limited presence in the computing fields is the dual stream theory of visual attention (McIntosh & Schenk, 2009). The dual stream theory of visual attention purports that global and local streams have separate yet integrated functions. The "global" stream that rapidly processes an entire scene and a "local" stream that processes details (Atkinson, 2017; Fink et al., 1997; Grinter et al., 2010; Vision, 1985). The integration of these two streams is paramount to the processing of the constant flow of visual input. The integration of the global and local streams is believed to be disrupted in autism, resulting in local interference (Rinehart et al., 2000a; Song & Hakoda, 2015; Wang et al., 2007). However local interference is not unique to autism. For some people with neurodivergence such as learning disabilities, dyslexia, autism, and ADHD, the integration of these two streams can be disrupted by a tendency to prioritize details (local) over the "big picture" (global) (Courchesne & Pierce, 2005; Foxton et al., 2003; Franceschini et al., 2017; Gargaro et al., 2018; Goldstein-Marcusohn et al., 2020; Gross, 2005; Guy et al., 2016; Hill et al., 2014; Imbir, 2019; Katagiri et al., 2013; Rinehart et al., 2000a). Likewise, local interference is not *always* found in autism research (Hayward et al., 2018). Most recently, a third pathway has been located that "computes the actions of moving faces and bodies (e.g., expressions, eye-gaze, audio-visual integration, intention, and mood) "(Pitcher & Ungerleider, 2021), social stimuli are addressed in Chap. 6. Regardless, these complex processes are not part of the design process in technology and warrants consideration.

Global processing is the processing of a holistic understanding of an object, event, or scene (e.g., seeing a forest before seeing the trees). By perceiving the whole, a person gets a sense of the structure of a stimulus—the holistic view. Local processing provides an understanding of the parts or details of a stimulus and has been referred to as analytic processing. These hierarchical processes are delegated to different sensory neuronal pathways, creating two separate streams of information. Global processing is presumed to occur automatically and preconscious while local processing is hypothesized to be processed more slowly and consciously (Bouvet et al., 2011; Norman, 2002). The global pathway is often described as faster than the local pathway, and this is hypothesized to be because the global pathway processes load average spatial frequencies whereas the local pathway processes higher spatial frequencies which takes longer because of the additional detail (Bouvet et al., 2011) (Fig. 5.1).

Low Spatial Frequency   High Spatial Frequency

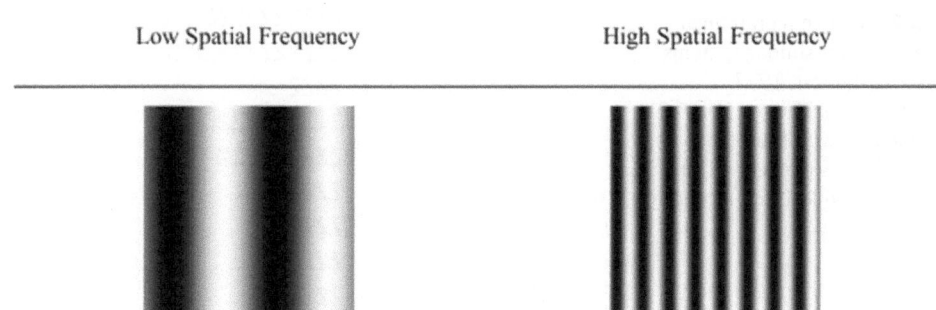

Fig. 5.1 Illustration of low and high spatial frequency. Spatial frequency vertical bars on the left show two black bars and two white bars equally spaced with some blur between them. The change in signal from one to the other is larger than the image on the right where there are within the same space, eight black vertical bars alternated with white bars. Here the signal is four times as high and the transition between black and white is crisper than the low spatial frequency example that is fuzzy at the transition point

The global precedence effect is important for (assistive) technology designers to understand because they decide what visual information gets translated into a technology and without an awareness of the separate global and local streams one level may be left out or tangled up together. Therefore, designers are encouraged to consider how global and local levels of information relate to sensory perception and therefore to assistive technology design.

Different stimulus features of an object or scene recruit one of the two levels of processing (McIntosh & Schenk, 2009; Vision, 1985). Global features are differentiated by visual receptors that are specialized to detect the overall shape, proximity to other stimuli, and movement. Local processing involves discerning the details. The Gestalt principles reflected in interface design leverage human perception of wholes to support the structure of an interface. Gestalt principles of continuity and proximity that are used when grouping objects (Graham, 2008; Han & Humphreys, 1999; Staudinger et al., 2011) leverage these assumptions to communicate the structure of an interface. The parts of an image support the function through the details (e.g., the details of an icon provide an indication of the function of a computer application). The global and local streams of information become integrated during cognitive processing to produce a complete mental representation of the stimuli. The stimuli themselves have features that may recruit one or both levels or types of processing, although cognitive neuroscientists continue to debate if this occurs in succession or in parallel (Bullier, 2001; McIntosh & Schenk, 2009; Norman, 2002).

When global processing is completed first in the sequence, it is known as *global precedence*. That is to say that global information is received first then processes local details as they are deemed relevant (i.e., global to local progression (Norman, 2002). In cognitive neuroscience research, ambiguous tasks and images are used to discern one's precedence. For example, when looking at an incongruent image (where local details are inconsistent

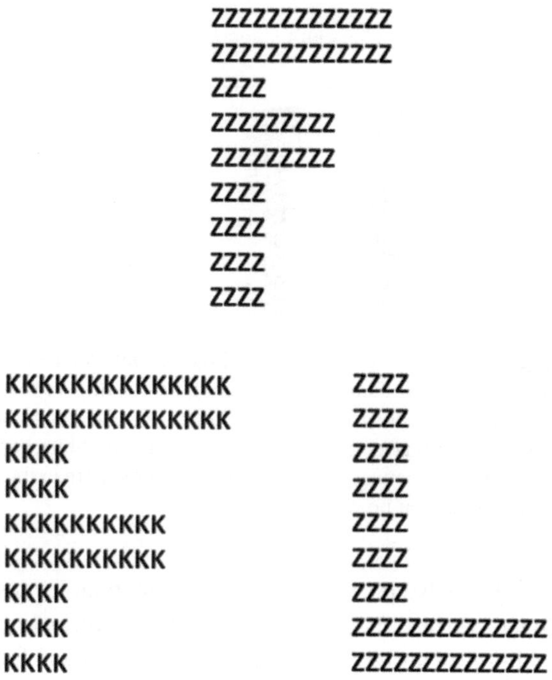

Fig. 5.2 Sample hierarchical
figures that are similar to items
on the Navon test, 1977
(Navon, 1977). The top item is
the target. The bottom items
are the choices to choose from
when a person is asked to find
the match

```
ZZZZZZZZZZZZZ
ZZZZZZZZZZZZZ
ZZZZ
ZZZZZZZZZ
ZZZZZZZZZ
ZZZZ
ZZZZ
ZZZZ
ZZZZ
```

```
KKKKKKKKKKKKKK        ZZZZ
KKKKKKKKKKKKKK        ZZZZ
KKKK                  ZZZZ
KKKK                  ZZZZ
KKKKKKKKKK            ZZZZ
KKKKKKKKKK            ZZZZ
KKKK                  ZZZZ
KKKK                  ZZZZZZZZZZZZZZ
KKKK                  ZZZZZZZZZZZZZZ
```

with global features) such as the top image in Fig. 5. 2, if a person selects the image on the bottom left to be the best match for the top image, that is an indication of a global precedence, whereas the image on the right is an indication of a local precedence. Global precedence is often assumed to be the primary processing style of most people (Navon, 1969, 1977, 1981), however, this is not the case for all people. Furthermore, precedence can be influenced by the immediate context. The task type can provide instruction about what to attend to (e.g., priming of the stimuli). The size of stimulus (e.g. visual angle) (Lamb & Robertson, 1990), the person's mood (Baumann & Kuhl, 2005; Chen et al., 2019; de Fockert & Cooper, 2014) all impact which type of processing is employed. In general, race (McKone et al., 2010) and culture (Davidoff et al., 2008) also impact precedence, as do changes over the lifespan (Scailquin, 2000; Staudinger et al., 2011). What is important is that a person has access to both levels or types of information and can integrate them when needed. Lastly, as researchers have found that training a global to local progression, reading skills in children with reading difficulties can improve (Franceschini et al., 2017). Therefore, this chapter explores a digital filter to manipulate the presentation of scenes to promote a global to local progression.

Local Interference in Autism

Many studies have found that people with autism display a local visual preference (Goldstein-Marcusohn et al., 2020; Kaliukhovich et al., 2021; Katagiri et al., 2013; Rinehart et al., 2000b). However, when a local preference becomes *local interference* (i.e., integration of global and local streams is interrupted) this leads to atypical visual perception, cognition, and communication (Behrmann et al., 2006; Chawarska & Shic, 2009; Robertson & Baron-Cohen, 2017). Visual Perception requires (at least) two streams that smoothly integrate a global (dorsal) and local (ventral) information over time (Badcock et al., 2005; Bouvet et al., 2011; Deruelle et al., 2004; Hughes et al., 1996; Vision, 1985). However, that is not the case in autism and other developmental disorders (Grinter et al., 2010). In autism, local processing is intact but may become backlogged in the higher order processing when increased complexity is added to forming a gist (Bertone et al., 2005; Grinter et al., 2010; Guy et al., 2016; Robertson & Baron-Cohen, 2017). Complex stimuli require global processing and a precedence for local processing in autism has been demonstrated with social and non-social stimuli (Behrmann et al., 2006).

Linking Low-Level Features to Global Content in Natural Scenes

The global and local visual pathways serve different functions. The global pathway is dedicated to tracking and controlling movement while the local pathway analyzes features to determine for identification (Norman, 2002). The visual system splits functions for processing low-level vision–such as color, luminance, and spatial frequency, see Fig. 5.1 for illustration of spatial frequency. Low levels are processed globally (Hughes et al., 1990; Oliva & Schyns, 1997). Luminance contrast and visual texture (i.e., spatial frequency) both support global form detection (Badcock et al., 2005; Silvestre et al., 2020). A specific range of spatial frequency that correlates to the physical world (nature, not created digitally). Natural images are processed globally first (Hübner, 1997; Hughes et al., 1990, 1996; Kihara & Takeda, 2019; Lamb & Yund, 1996; Shulman et al., 1986). These visual perception factors have been linked to poor outcomes in learning—specifically the reduction of visual attention to low spatial frequency for autistic people (Bertone et al., 2005; de Jong et al., 2008; Deruelle et al., 2004; Koh et al., 2010).

Luminance also is perceived across two streams as local luminance (first-order pathway) and local contrast (Badcock et al., 2005). Higher luminance draws the eye early in visual processing, see Fig. 5.3 for illustration of luminance. Vision research confirms this and adds an additional pathway that detects decrements to luminance (Badcock et al., 2005). Machine learning research has revealed that the visual attention of participants with autism was not only at the local level (as opposed to global) but even tended towards a hyper-local, pixel-level visual attention (Wang et al., 2015; Xu et al., 2014). Pixel-level differences warrant a deeper analysis of the roles of global and local neural mechanisms in

Low Luminance   High Luminance

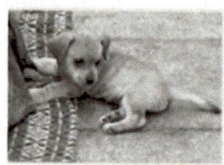   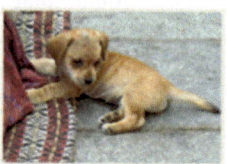

Fig. 5.3 Illustration of luminance. On the left is an image with low luminance which appears as a grayscale image. On the right there is the same picture with high luminance and in full color. Luminance and chroma are highly correlated therefore affecting one directly affects the other

local interference. For autistic people, however, local interference, or the tendency to prioritize local details at the cost the whole, can create a wide variety of academic challenges (Bullen et al., 2022; Stevenson, n.d.) and social challenges (see (Rinehart et al., 2000a) for summary). These sensory-level insights have not been applied to assistive technology beyond the lab.

Eye Movement as a Metric of Visual Attention

Eye gaze is considered a proxy for visual attention (Liechty et al., 2003) in autism research and has been considered a "potential porthole into the current cognitive processes" (John & Theo Engell-Nielsen, 1995). Several aspects of eye gaze behavior have been explored in autism research, especially, eye gaze fixation (aka fixations), saccades, and eye gaze path. Another eye gaze metric is the dilation of the pupil via pupillometry. Dilation of the pupil is used as a proxy for arousal level during viewing. This chapter is focused only on overt eye gaze behaviors. Eye gaze has been classified as overt and covert attention (Liechty et al., 2003) meaning that the observable eye movement data is the overt thus a measurable metric that overlaps significantly with the hidden, covert mental attention of the viewer. Thus, understanding the function of different eye gaze behaviors helps researchers draw conclusions about a viewer's attention and emotional state.

Eye Gaze Path

Eye gaze path refers to the areas the eye has traveled during viewing, see Fig. 5.4. Eye gaze paths have been less employed as a metric because they are idiosyncratic and depend on personal experience in terms of how someone orients to an image, however in this work it could be of interest if the filtering changes the path toward the hot spots. it is less of a concern where someone starts and ends their viewing but rather if they span the whole image to cover the areas of Interest and if they do that early on in viewing, see Fig. 5.4 of eye pathways example.

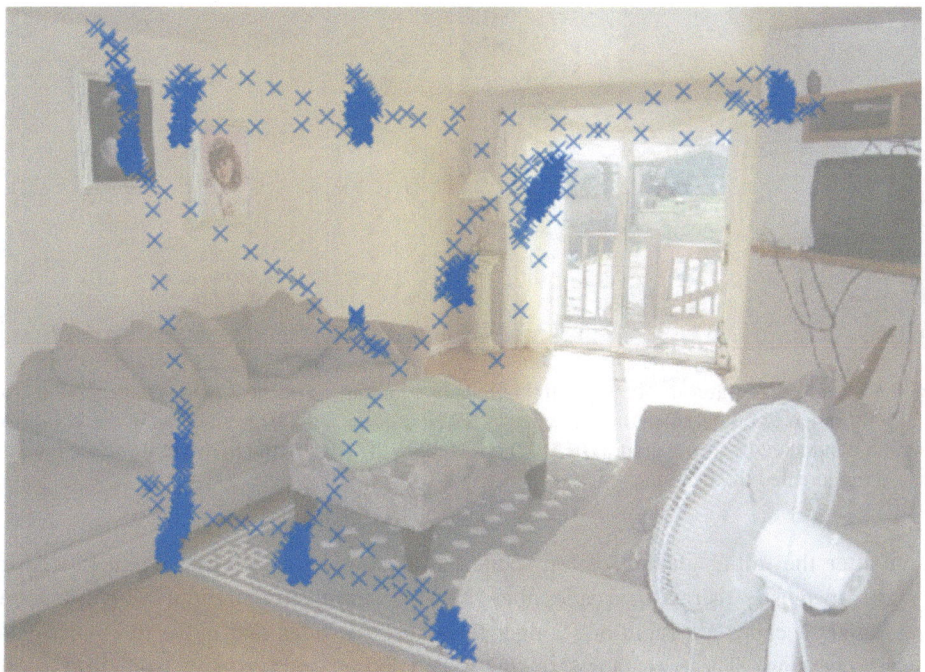

Fig. 5.4 Example of Eye Gaze Path for 3 s of viewing by a 40-year-old autistic man in an eye tracking system with capture rate of 1000 Hz

Eye fixations refer to a cluster of eye gaze points in a similar area. Eye gaze occurs several times a second, and only areas that are viewed over time are processed at the local level. Therefore, fixations are a metric of where foveal vision has occurred (Rayner, 1998). Covert visual attention at least as we can see things perfectly as well. This metric is used most frequently in research in terms of frequency and duration regarding areas of interest in an image or video. Many software packages included in eye tracking systems have their own algorithms for detecting fixations that are based on a combination of features from proximity of the points from each other and duration. The fixations used to determine the neurotypical heat maps in this work were calculated using an open source– Cluster Fixation (König & Buffalo, 2014).

Saccades

Saccades are the rapid eye movements from one area to another between eye gaze fixation (Salvucci & Goldberg, 2000). During saccades, vision is "essential suppressed" during saccades (Liechty et al., 2003). Depending on the speed and duration of the movement are believed to indicate different types of processing (i.e., global which is also called ambient and local which is also called foveal). A transition from global to local is expected to

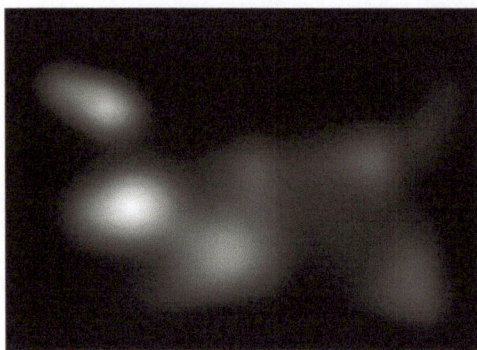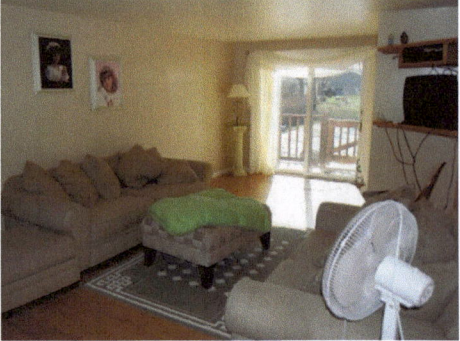

Fig. 5.5 Regions of Interests shown as light areas of heatmaps. This heat map was generated from an algorithm based on 3 s of natural viewing by 20 Neurotypical College students in the USA from research conducted by Wang et al. (2015). The image on the right is the living room scene that was viewed that created the heat map

occur after the initial glazing of the scene has occurred. In general, global processing is made up mostly of rapid saccades that span the stimuli to determine where to focus, thus initial saccades are rapid and longer than later saccades that move to collect detail (local processing). These saccades are slower and shorter as they move from a focus area to nearby focus area. Some researchers claim the global process occurs during the early phase of viewing (within the first 2 s) of natural viewing (Ito et al. 2017; Srikantharajah & Ellard, 2022).

Regions of Interests

A region of interest is an area on an image or in a video that is the target of the researcher's work. Generally, eye tracking studies for research or marketing purposes are interested in knowing where people look or predicting where they might look, see Fig. 5.5. Regions of interest in natural images (not staged for advertisement or digitally rendered by a human) usually draw the eye to social content (e.g., people, living things). Natural scenes make up much of the visual input humans take in and human eyes are designed to rapidly perceive the natural world based on low-level visual features (Hughes et al., 1996). In this work, it is the neurotypical hotspots that are employed as a representation of the global processing of image as saccades three the eyes to the areas that are then fixated upon.

Technologies from Top Down and Bottom Up

One project supports global processing by systematically teaching visual attention to a whole image by differentially rewarding correct answers. Selectively attending to parts of images is termed stimulus overselectivity (Lovaas et al., 1971; Ploog, 2010). The

GoGoGames iPad game targets skills training to reduce overselectivity (i.e., an observable behavior due to local interference) (Boyd et al., 2017; Hiniker et al., 2013), but no technology simply provides immediate access to global information of visual content. Another project that is the most closely related to this proposed work is the half static video project (Lee et al., 2016) in which the researchers freeze the background of the video while permitting the main objects to continue in motion allowing for the focus to be directed to the most salient pieces. This related work directly addresses the local interference problem. However, at this moment the approach lacks automation and scalability. Lastly, my work has attempted to address bottom-up processes to change to output.

Features of stimuli that draw one's attention are considered salient. Visual salience is impacted by the purpose of viewing as visual attention is influenced by both sensory perception and cognitive functioning. Visual attention is a bridge between sensory processing and cognitive processing. As visual processing interacts with both low-level processing of sensory information and high-level processing of cognitive information it is in between these two processes that visual attention occurs and reoccurs. Therefore, visual tension is used as a metric to understand how people are receiving sensory information but more often how they are processing information cognitively. Visual attention has a long history of being the focus of autism as differences have been noted for several decades as mentioned in the introduction.

Even though visual attention is a bridge between sensory and cognitive processes, research has explored both of these approaches in the search for explanations for the visual attention differences in some people with autism. From the cognitive processing perspective, the low amounts of attention to people in many research studies on autism has been attributed to difficulties processing emotion. What is fascinating is that even within these studies discussing high level processing of emotion there is also a connection to low level sensory processing as the input is first received by the senses in the form of low-level information. Higher spatial frequency has been associated with local detail processing whereas lower spatial frequency gives way to form and pattern perception (Ellemberg et al., 1999), however both high and low spatial frequencies code the structure of an image (Shulman et al., 1986; Shulman & Wilson, 1987).

An example of low-level, sensory level processing that is frequently related to high level face processing is spatial frequency. It has been found that low level spatial frequency is processed by the global system whereas high level special frequency is processed by the local system. As the global system has been indicated as slower in integrating the local details in autism, this has implications for face processing. For example, this specific difference in autism in attention-based gaze shifts have been found to be influenced by the emotional content which requires higher order cognitive processing of a scene and its spatial frequency which requires low level sensory processing (de Jong et al., 2008). This phenomenon reflects the relation between sensory processing and cognitive processing.

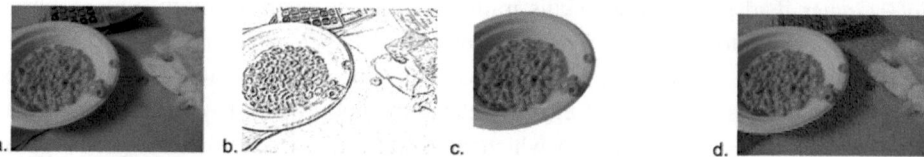

Fig. 5.6 Low fidelity filter options along with baseline image: **a** Baseline, **b** Lined drawing, **c** White background, **d** Gray blur background. These 4 types were put together as a GIF for a 5th filter. Each of the filter options employs a different way to manipulate the spatial frequency and luminance in an image to promote processing the global information which in this image is the bowl of cereal

Therefore, a person's sensory processing style impacts one's visual attention. Subsequently, people with autism may use spatial frequency differently (Koh et al., 2010). Given this nuance, that these levels are both intact and are used preferentially by autistic people, improvement in global perception is feasible (Baisa et al., 2019).

Global Filter Project

In the Global Filter work, previous research provides eye gaze of neurotypical adults to assist children with autism with global to local visual attention(Wang et al., 2015; Xu et al., 2014). This technology aimed to support autistic children—a work-around to local interference by manipulating sensory input. The hypothesis in the Global Filter project was that by visually-highlighting the global features to shift visual attention to globally-relevant areas in a scene, the global filter will reduce the distracting features of the image that are believed to be the cause of local interference–thus allowing the participants to utilize these hints and see the whole image or the big picture. Several iterations of designs were tested with children with autism, see Fig. 5.6 for low fidelity prototypes of the global filter.

Low Fidelity Design Probes

To create the filter, images were digitally manipulated by desaturating and blurring non-relevant detail as determined by heat maps collected for a set of previously studied images. In previous research the heatmaps were used to make an algorithm based on the aggregation of 15 Neurotypical young adults to predict where people look in natural viewing conditions (Wang et al., 2015; Xu et al., 2014). Fifty images were digitally manipulated using a filter designed with extensive collaboration with the field site clinicians. Eleven autistic children with autism who display developmental language delay tested the system and their eye tracking data was compared. The main question was if the eye tracking behavior differed significantly between the baseline and filtered images. Findings revealed that this group of children performed well in the baseline condition as well as in the filtered condition. The impact of the filter is difficult to discern as there was not much room to improve given the score of 1.49 out of 2 shows an average that is higher than an average local score of 1. In one of two sessions they performed about the same in both conditions and in the second session the group performed slower with the filter. Individual cases reveal patterns in eye tracking that vary by day and/or condition. A deeper analysis is required to draw conclusions of the utility and further work is needed to discern the efficacy of such a tool.

To understand how a user might take in an augmented image for the purpose of highlighting the global information, four prototypes were made to expand Explorer different theories that might make for good designs. The first is using a black and white line drawing to minimize the Shadows call this the black and white filter the second is just to completely remove the background and leave it white so only the main object or objects appear in an image in the last is to pixelate and desaturated image so that high contrast areas and non-relevant regions are less salient and then the last option was to put these same filters together as a gift to promote a global to local progression.

The *line drawing filter* changes the entire image to a black and white line drawing that emphasizes the shape of objects and boundaries between them. This filter also removes high spatial-frequency sections such as shading thus reducing the image to shapes of objects as the shape is processed by the global stream (Oliva & Schyns, 1997), see Fig. 5.6b. To make images appear as line drawings, the spatial frequency was set at a consistent level across the whole image, rather than varying for contours or high-contrast areas. For this purpose, commercial filters were used that uniformly affected the whole image rather than specific features to reduce sensory input. The lined drawing filter produced images inspired by icons that are commonly used in Augmentative and Alternative Communication systems (AAC) that present objects as line drawings (Ganz et al., 2015) for people who do not communicate verbally–however the images in this study still contained background information. It was hypothesized that the line drawings resulted in a simplified image that could promote global processing because all features that could be processed locally were removed (color, depth, movement, shadows) leaving only the course, spatial information of sketch-like objects, potentially enabling learning through more efficient visual processing of global information (Oliva & Schyns, 1997). Shadows have been shown to interfere with object recognition for many autistic children (Becchio et al., 2010). Therefore, the line drawing filter was designed to support recognition of key objects based on the shape and location rather than color or shading (Becchio et al., 2010; Oliva & Schyns, 1997).

The *white background filter* highlights the image's primary object(s) by retaining the original color and shading and removing the background, see Fig. 5.6c. The background for the primary object is white space with the primary objects differentiated algorithmically (Lu & Guo, 1999). It was hypothesized that a primary object with a white background could promote global processing because irrelevant local information has been removed. This approach assumes that the object-centered approach (Fink et al., 1997), by supporting the identification of one or more prominent objects, may be sufficient to activate a schema of the scene, and thus facilitate recognition (Oliva & Torralba, 2002). As with the line drawing filter, this approach is also common in AAC systems and low-tech material used therapeutically for communication training (Light et al., 2019).

The *gray blur filter* presents the primary objects with their original color and shading, against a greyscale blurred background, see Fig. 5.6d. This filter highlights the main object while preserving but diminishing the background. This scene-centered approach (Oliva & Torralba, 2002) stems from the notion that by removing some local features of the scene (e.g., color and smoothing the transitions between pixels), enough information is still present to reliably estimate the global information of the scene by providing some information of the environment (i.e., "context frame" (Bar, 2004)). This technique resembles the blurred background that has become popular in video conferencing apps that are optional for those who wish to hide their environment or view a screen with less distraction. In the case of video conferencing, however, the producer of the content chooses to use this filter. In the case of an access technology using such a filter, the content consumer would need to be able to turn on such a filter.

The animation filter is a 3 s GIF that presents varying levels of global information to mimic the typical global to local progression. The GIF showed the global object(s) with white background first (core objects), followed by the blurred image (hint of context), then the raw image (full image) is a low-fidelity attempt to simulate the global-to-local progression, where global information is processed first then integrated with local information (Ahissar & Hochstein, 2004). This process is believed to occur as neurons are specialized and geographically localized to process certain features (e.g., movement, color) (Previc, 1990). In the case of autistic visual attention, the global processing neurons are thought to be intact when employed in isolation but overridden by the undifferentiated details. By activating global neurons first without local interference (as intended with the white background filter), then adding context back in using hypothesized global strategies (line drawing to blurred to raw), this filter aims to create an evolving context and eventually the complete raw picture. The animation aspect was intended to give the global stream an advantage in prioritizing details without interference of all the details.

In a field study, 20 autistic children viewed 50 unique images for 3 s each. Of the 5 conditions, 10 images per condition, results indicated the filtered images with white background provided the most global verbal responses ($p = 0.003$) and gray blurred background also producing significant results, $p = 0.03$. These results indicate visually differentiating core elements from irrelevant elements in a scene is necessary to reduce sensory local interference [manuscript in submission]. This insight goes beyond simply reducing the *amount of sensory* input to directly indicating *which details are critical* from noncritical. By highlighting critical elements, top-down processing has been simulated. The proof of concept had been established through the immediate, observable change in verbal response. The next target was to compare verbal output and eye gaze behavior in 11 other autistic children.

High Fidelity Prototype

To create a functioning prototype of a high-fidelity filter, hot spots from heat maps were used to determine regions of interest to compare the durations of eye fixations. The hot spots were from an open-source eye prediction model based on aggregated heatmaps of neurotypical viewers (Huang et al., 2015; Jiang et al., 2015). The initial seconds of neurotypical viewing for global processing to operationalize regions of interest. Regions of interest in this work were areas of an image containing global content as a scan to understand the gist of an image is believed to occur within the first few seconds of viewing (Fink et al., 1997). Therefore, the early viewing fixation data can be used to generate the hotspots to indicate global elements at the first moment of viewing. In the corresponding experiment with 11 autistic children, I demonstrated that manipulating low level features of non-salient areas support eye gaze shift to the salient areas. Findings from scoring video of eye gaze viewing revealed a differential effect of luminance and spatial frequency (Boyd et al., 2022). This work serves as a proof of concept of feasibility to direct eye gaze to salient areas through the manipulation of the luminance, color, and spatial frequency of non-relevant local features areas (Boyd et al., 2022; Cibrian et al., 2020; Sean et al., 2019). The high-fidelity insights drove the rationale for making global areas more salient.

In the second iteration of the high-fidelity filter, the contrast was intensified to create a larger difference in low-level visual characteristics between the salient and non-salient features and measured the duration of fixations with a screen-based eye tracker, see Fig. 5.7. Findings presented in the student's undergraduate thesis paper (Mody, 2022) revealed that the neurotypical participants were 8% more likely to fixate in a global hotspot than the neurodiverse group. The neurotypical group also demonstrated significantly longer fixation durations in global hotspots (average duration = 123 ms longer, $p < 0.01$) in both conditions (baseline and filtered) from the neurodiverse group. The neurodiverse group produced less consistent findings as a group, however one participant demonstrated longer fixation durations (33 ms longer, $p < 0.01$) in filtered condition; providing evidence that the filter had the desired impact on eye gaze in some individuals.

User experience data also confirmed that the filtered images may reduce visual processing burden. For example, one autistic participant in (Mody, 2022) was unable to maintain calibration with the eye tracker as she could not look at the calibration point long enough for the computer program to recognize her eye gaze points (3 s), this can be due to vision problems. She was asked to state "what the picture was about" for a handful of the images. She was shown the raw image and asked what the image was about, she said "container", and when she was shown the filtered image, she said "pantry," see Fig. 5.7. This indicates a shift towards global processing since the container is a small, single object, a local detail, and the pantry is the big picture, the global idea. She also mentioned that the "black and white" images, filtered images, were "easier to look at" because "you don't have to focus that hard."

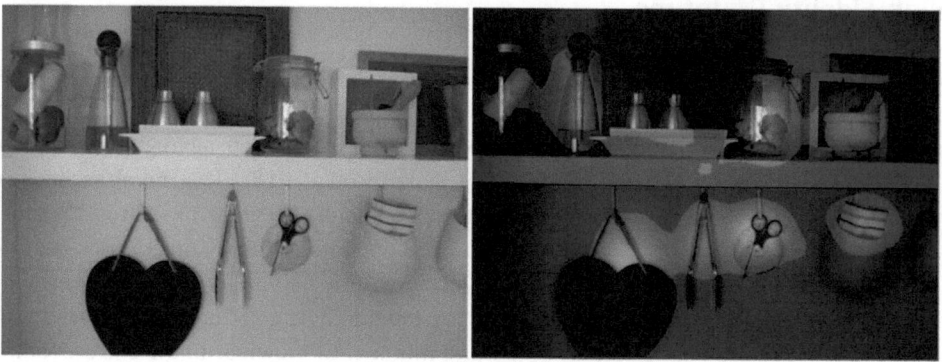

Fig. 5.7 The raw image on the left, Experimental filtered image on the right. Images and heatmaps of aggregated hotspots from neurotypical participants were gathered from an open-source dataset at (Wang et al., 2015)

PART 2: Hidden Hierarchy in Augmented and Alternative Communication Systems

Sensory perception is linked to all language domains, including phonology, morphology, syntax, semantics, and pragmatics (Kamio et al., 2007). These domains include phonology (speech sound system), syntax (sentence structure, grammar), semantics (word meanings) and pragmatics (social use of language). This work is concerned with the lexical-semantic processing that is frequently reported as a disorder in autism. Autistic individuals have demonstrated atypical lexical-semantic processing in semantic decision tasks (Kamio et al., 2007) and as measured by Event Related Potentials (ERPs) in a picture-word matching paradigm (Cantiani et al., 2016). Lexical-semantic processing refers to our ability to assign meaning (label) to an object or experience in our environment. For example, a child learns the word *dog* by perceiving multiple dogs in their environment over time until that term is represented in their lexicon (i.e., internal dictionary).

As a child acquires more experiences with differing features (auditory-sound of a bark, visual motor-playing fetch) their semantic representation of *dog* becomes more robust. According to language theory, in an embodied language comprehension framework, lexical-semantic representation is directly linked to one's perceptions and real-world experiences with the label (Glenberg & Kaschak, 2002; Van Dam et al., 2010). For instance, participants perform lexical decision tasks more rapidly when a congruent action (e.g. moving the hand toward the mouth for "cup") is presented rather than an incongruent action (e.g. moving the hand away from the body) (Glenberg & Kaschak, 2002; Van Dam et al., 2010). Thus, the formation of lexical-semantic representation is based upon sensory perception abilities and experiences with the label such as how it looks, sounds, feels, tastes, and moves. In essence, the two constructs are inextricably connected. Specifically, basic sensory perception skills may constrain the development of robust lexical-semantic representations needed for higher-level language skills, and these in turn, shape lower-level perceptions (Cantiani et al., 2016).

The ability to process and visually attend to objects and events in our environment is important to the acquisition of higher-order language, and for autistic individuals, differences in global visual processing may hinder their ability to develop higher-level lexical-semantic representations that are more efficient and substantiated. Lower-level processes such as sensory perception and movement matter–they are not simply automatic, involuntary processes that are from our prehistoric brains. Rather, perceiving perceptual features (visual, auditory, tactile, motor) are critical to the understanding and embodiment of cognition and language.

AAC and Autism

Sensory perception, particularly visual perception, in autistic people has been found to overly rely on details rather than default to perceiving stimuli as a whole unit, termed *local interference* (Courchesne & Pierce, 2005; Guy et al., 2016; Nayar et al., 2017). Local interference is intertwined with, and demonstrated through, communication. Complex language, such as expressing the main idea, is important, so integrating the local with the global is necessary for one to be able to see the "big picture" (global).

The focus on details of local interference negatively impacts linguistic abilities (Jolliffe & Baron-Cohen, 1999, 2000). For example, any individual with a language disorder, not specific to ASD, may experience challenges in comprehension and use of figurative language (Gernsbacher & Pripas-Kapit, 2012). Part of interpreting figurative language involves the integration of details into a whole as well as making inferences about information. Global processing is essential in the development of communication and is deeply rooted in more global forms of language, such as being able to understand (receptive) and use metaphors, paradoxes and oxymorons (expressive) (Beekman, 2019).

Receptive and expressive language are impacted not only by the interaction between sensory perception and lexical-semantic processing, but also by AAC use and design. The use of AAC can not only provide a means of expressive communication but also aid in receptive language abilities and overall language development (Dada et al., 2020; Romski et al., 2015; Rose et al., 2020). Sensory processing plays a role in facilitating expressive language because most AAC devices require the perception of visual symbols; therefore, for individuals with ASD who require AAC, the differences in sensory processing styles, the lexical-semantic processing challenges in conjunction with the constraints of AAC devices, impact the ability to generate and comprehend more abstract language. When an AAC device is designed with a focus on mostly basic functional responses (i.e., details, local forms), individuals are in turn, limited in their ability to communicate complex forms of language when needed, which ultimately leads to a narrowed learning experience.

Given the complexity of communication concerns in ASD, AAC interfaces need to establish a balance among multiple features and processes. Evidence-based practices for ASD and AAC focus on use of symbols, visual supports, voice output, and inclusion that are exemplified in some communication computer applications (Sennott & Bowker, 2009). Visual perceptual features such as symbol color, spatial arrangement, shape, and orientation should be considered in the AAC design process (Wilkinson & Jagaroo, 2004), as well as specific symbol organizations that contribute to efficient visual searching, as found for children with developmental disabilities (Wilkinson & Madel, 2019). Design decisions often optimize speed and efficiency over complexity of language expression, as an AAC device may only have one choice of the word readily available to select. Thus, the affordances of the AAC are subject to device constraints. Essentially, the natural speech modality affords more global communication opportunities and diversity of expression when compared to the AAC modality. Functional local details are frequently the only efficient options to convey higher order, complex lexical-semantic representations. Thus, individuals who require AAC experience increased processing loads as they must visually process a scene in their environment and then generate the visual memory or a visual search strategy to identify the target icon on their device. Additionally, the semantic content of the visual scene impacts processing speed and efficiency.

Semantic salience is a feature that precedes conscious comprehension. Human figures in photographs are particularly noticeable in capturing visual attention (Wilkinson & Light, 2011; Wilkinson & Light, 2014). Semantic content is processed rapidly with local details integrated over time (Campana et al., 2016; Robertson & Baron-Cohen, 2017). Visual salience refers to the intensity of the visual aspects of an image as opposed to the semantic salience of an image that would regard the meaning of the image and is also critical for those with slower semantic processing. As would be inferred, the structure provided by low-level visual elements matter in the environment and on the AAC device. Research on visual scene displays has found that design features such as placement of a navigation bar influenced visual attention to meaningful elements in the scene, highlighting the influence of design on processing of semantic content (O'Neill et al., 2019).

Directions for Augmentative and Alternative Communication Design for Local Interference

For autistic people who use AAC, the designs of AAC devices can extend opportunities to enhance language processing, but also may constrain communication in efforts to promote functionality. This study explored assistive technology design features that could support language processing through manipulation of visual attention to promote global expressive language output. Results indicated that the presence of visual filters had the potential to enhance performance for individuals who required AAC and autistic people that used natural speech. Furthermore, item difficulty and discrimination indices were important to evaluating visual and semantic salience. Finally, collaboration between disciplines is critical to answer these complex, important questions.

Future studies could target access to more robust conversational language using AAC, design could be considered both for input sensory perception adaptations (i.e., visual attention) and output support for the interface design. In other words, global filter automation could support language processing for students with developmental disabilities who require assistive technology to promote more robust communication. Future research in technology design could promote global-first responding through filters and providing details systematically. Pre-processing an image to visually highlight global features could benefit students with developmental disabilities who use natural speech as well as those who require assistive technology. For example, using algorithms that predict the initial eye gaze in neurotypical viewers (Xu et al., 2014) could provide the conditions needed to filter global from local details as seen in Fig. 5.8.

Then, machine vision could process global details to provide text options related to those areas; therefore, global filter automation could create a novel assistive technology to support receptive as well as expressive communication as seen in Fig. 5.5. Employing

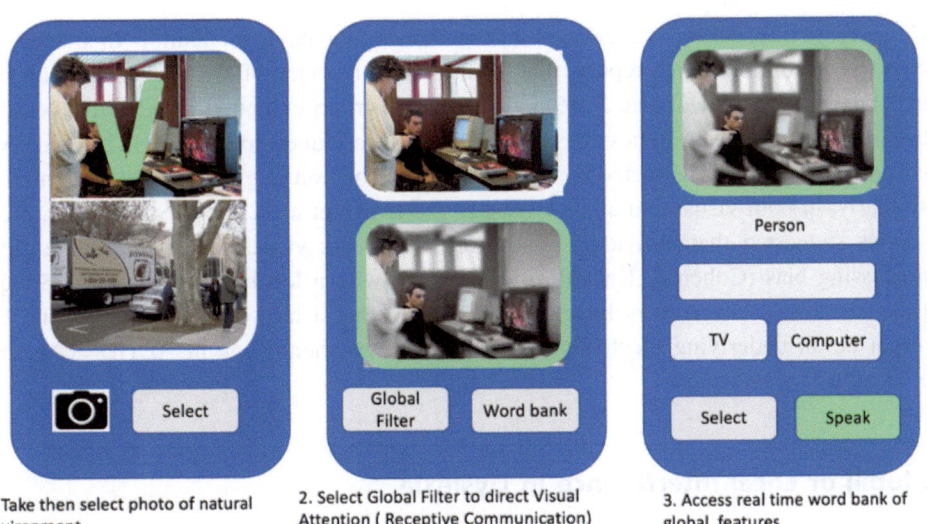

Fig. 5.8 Low Fidelity Mockup of global semantic filter for AAC. Three screens of user interaction with a novel assistive technology to filter images for receptive and expressive support. On the first screen, a user would select an image. On the second screen, a user would select semantic filter mode. On the third screen, a user would select words from a word bank provided for semantic features

both receptive and expressive supports in a single device may aid those with language processing challenges regardless of communication modality.

Local Interference Beyond Autism

Regarding visual attention specifically, many neurodivergent conditions are linked to specific difficulties with accessing one or the other style of processing. For example, dyslexia is associated with difficulty reading from either analyzing letters or seeing words as whole units, which requires local and global processing (Goldstein-Marcusohn et al., 2020). People with Attention Deficit Hyperactivity disorder (ADHD) demonstrate challenges with processing the whole picture (Helenius et al., 2011). Those with obsessive–compulsive disorder focus on detail (Yovel et al., 2005). Those with autism may be "disinclined" (Koldewyn et al., 2013) to attend to global features and may engage in the overselectivity of local details. Though the above examples involve visual perception, the same patterns of differences in gestalt (global) processing have been observed regarding auditory and tactile perception (Conway & Christiansen, 2005).

Local Interference in ADHD

Contrary to the DSM-5 description of ADHD as not paying attention to details, the NAVON in some research reports that local interference/lack of a global bias is observed in ADHD (Song & Hakoda, 2015). "The ADHD group exhibited no global processing bias, indicating similar processing for global and local dimensions, implying that individuals with ADHD are distracted by incongruent information in global and local conditions similarly, in both visual and auditory tasks" (Akerman et al., 2023). "Specifically, recent studies suggested that individuals with ADHD process visual scenes without a global processing bias (Cohen & Kalanthroff, 2019), or with a local processing bias (Song & Hakoda, 2015). Researchers have even suggested that a lack of global processing bias might be an underlying mechanism of a few known phenomena in ADHD" (Akerman et al., 2023).

Global or Local Interference in Dyslexia

Dyslexia is complicated in that studies continue to show mixed results. Some of this complexity is due to the multiple abilities required such as visual attention, reading, and auditory processing. As "words are comprised of both global and local components and deficiencies in the different mechanisms can lead to a different profile of reading impairment. Deficiency in the local detailed processing could lead to more reading errors and deficiency in the general global processing could lead to speed reading impairment" (Goldstein-Marcusohn et al., 2020). Therefore, local and global interference are attributed to displaying dyslexia.

Global Interference has been observed in dyslexia where dyslexia research participants were faster than control at identifying impossible figures which require global processing (von Károlyi, 2001). Schneps et al. (2012) found that individuals with dyslexia perform better in a low-pass filtered natural scenes task in which the perception for low spatial frequency components is examined" (Goldstein-Marcusohn et al., 2020).

Local Interference in Other Neurodivergent Conditions

Lack of global bias/Local interference has been found in bipolar disorder as deficits in global movement processing across a variety of timescales (O'Bryan et al., 2014). Local Interference has also been indicated in Obsessive Compulsive Disorder (Yovel et al., 2005) and anxiety (Tyler & Tucker, 1982). Local Interference has been discovered in depression (de Fockert & Cooper, 2014) as well as in Body Dysmorphic Disorder (Wong et al., 2022). In summary, a number of neurodivergencies demonstrate local precedence and local interference. Some researchers have suggested that global to local training could be beneficial (Franceschini et al., 2017; Robertson & Baron-Cohen, 2017). Digital strategies to work around local interference via assistive technologies could benefit not only autistic people but a wider array of neurodivergencies.

Implications for Design

Visual Attention Layer of The Sensory Accommodation Framework provides an example of a global filter where local irrelevant information is filtered out and only local details that support the global gist of an image are presented to the user. In Fig. 5.9, Sensory input has traveled from the bottom of the cone all the way up to the visual attention layer. Here information is filtered to be more comprehensible. Global Information is allowed to pass through the filter where local information that does not contribute to the global information is blocked.

Designers of technologies are encouraged to consider these two streams of information especially when they must make decisions on how to capture stimuli in the physical world through a technology. Every variable has to be operationalized and parameters set. How this is done is not often transparent to the end user. What information is removed is not always explained either knowing that there is a hierarchy to visual information that will assist designers and making choices about what to include and what not to include. This may be obvious to someone who integrates local and global Information very well but for someone with local interference, having the global Information highlighted could save precious processing energy.

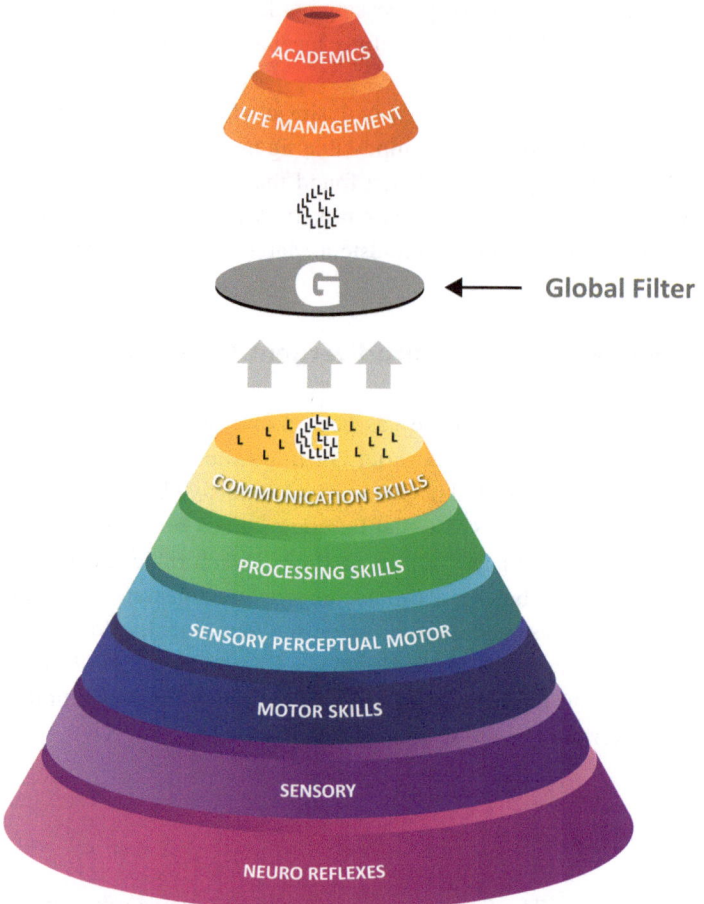

Fig. 5.9 Visual Attention Layer of The Sensory Accommodation Framework. At the visual attention layer in the learning cone sensory input is passing through in the form of global and local information. The little L's represent the local information and the Big G represents the collection of local details that create the global gist. Only the (local) details that are relevant to the gist pass through the global filter to create a global image consisting of local details

Conclusion

Because of the complex sensory experience, people with autism may be inclined to attend to local information over global information. This can be a strength or a challenge, depending on the task at hand (Robertson & Baron-Cohen, 2017). However, since much of the stimulation information in the world is occurring continuously (e.g., dynamically), being able to access Global Information eases the burden of processing every detail to determine what is the main detail by filtering out the relevant information to the gist of an image, the labor of relying on local processing over sluggish Global processing is theoretically alleviated. Additionally, a number of superior visual perceptual abilities exist among people with autism (Mottron et al., 2006). These strengths tend to lie in the local domain, therefore visuals used by a designer can be leveraged to assist with rapid visual processing of the gist and ongoing visual attention.

References

Abdo, M., & Al Osman, H. (2019). Technology impact on reading and writing skills of children with autism: A systematic literature review. *Health and Technology, 9*(5), 725–735. https://doi.org/10.1007/s12553-019-00317-4

Ahissar, M., & Hochstein, S. (2004). The reverse hierarchy theory of visual perceptual learning. *Trends in Cognitive Sciences, 8*(10), 457–464. https://doi.org/10.1016/j.tics.2004.08.011

Akerman, A., Etkovitch, A., & Kalanthroff, E. (2023). Global-local processing in ADHD is not limited to the visuospatial domain: Novel evidence from the auditory domain. *Journal of Attention Disorders*. https://doi.org/10.1177/10870547231153952

Almourad, M. B., & Bataineh, E. (2020). Visual Attention toward Human Face Recognizing for Autism Spectrum Disorder and Normal Developing Children: An Eye Tracking Study. In *Proceedings of the 2020 The 6th International Conference on E-Business and Applications* (pp. 99–104). https://doi.org/10.1145/3387263.3387283

Amso, D., Haas, S., Tenenbaum, E., Markant, J., & Sheinkopf, S. J. (2014). Bottom-up attention orienting in young children with autism. *Journal of Autism and Developmental Disorders, 44*(3), 664–673. https://doi.org/10.1007/s10803-013-1925-5

Atkinson, J. (2017). The Davida Teller Award Lecture, 2016: visual brain development: a review of "dorsal stream vulnerability"—motion, mathematics, amblyopia, actions, and attention. *Journal of Vision, 17*(3), 26. https://doi.org/10.1167/17.3.26

Badcock, D. R., Clifford, C. W. G., & Khuu, S. K. (2005). Interactions between luminance and contrast signals in global form detection. *Vision Research, 45*(7), 881–889. https://doi.org/10.1016/j.visres.2004.09.042

Baisa, A., Mevorach, C., & Shalev, L. (2019). Can performance in Navon letters among people with autism be affected by saliency? Reexamination of the literature. *Review journal of autism and developmental disorders, 6*, 1–12

Baisa, A., Mevorach, C., & Shalev, L. (2021). Hierarchical processing in ASD is driven by exaggerated salience effects, not local bias. *Journal of Autism and Developmental Disorders, 51*(2), 666–676. https://doi.org/10.1007/s10803-020-04578-1

Bar, M. (2004). Visual objects in context. *Nature Reviews Neuroscience, 5*(8), Article 8. https://doi.org/10.1038/nrn1476

Baumann, N., & Kuhl, J. (2005). Positive affect and flexibility: overcoming the precedence of global over local processing of visual information. *Motivation and Emotion, 29*(2), 123–134. https://doi.org/10.1007/s11031-005-7957-1

Becchio, C., Mari, M., & Castiello, U. (2010). Perception of shadows in children with autism spectrum disorders. *PLoS ONE, 5*(5), e10582. https://doi.org/10.1371/journal.pone.0010582

Beekman, L. M. (2019). Clearly misunderstood: The ambiguous language test for students with and without language disorders. [Case Western Reserve University]. https://etd.ohiolink.edu/acprod/odb_etd/etd/r/1501/10?clear=10&p10_accession_num=case1563362510636297

Behrmann, M., Thomas, C., & Humphreys, K. (2006). Seeing it differently: Visual processing in autism. *Trends in Cognitive Sciences, 10*(6), 258–264. https://doi.org/10.1016/j.tics.2006.05.001

Bertone, A., Mottron, L., Jelenic, P., & Faubert, J. (2005). Enhanced and diminished visuo-spatial information processing in autism depends on stimulus complexity. *Brain, 128*(10), 2430–2441. https://doi.org/10.1093/brain/awh561

Bouvet, L., Rousset, S., Valdois, S., & Donnadieu, S. (2011). Global precedence effect in audition and vision: Evidence for similar cognitive styles across modalities. *Acta Psychologica, 138*(2), 329–335. https://doi.org/10.1016/j.actpsy.2011.08.004

Boyd, L. E., Ringland, K. E., Faucett, H., Hiniker, A., Klein, K., Patel, K., & Hayes, G. R. (2017). Evaluating an iPad Game to Address Overselectivity in Preliterate AAC Users with Minimal Verbal Behavior. In *Proceedings of the 19th International ACM SIGACCESS Conference on Computers and Accessibility* (pp. 240–249). https://doi.org/10.1145/3132525.3132551

Boyd, L., Berardi, V., Hughes, D., Cibrian, F., Johnson, J., Sean, V., DelPizzo-Cheng, E., Mackin, B., Tusneem, A., Mody, R., Jones, S., & Lotich, K. (2022). Manipulating image luminance to improve eye gaze and verbal behavior in autistic children. *Humanities and Social Sciences Communications, 9*(1), Article 1. https://doi.org/10.1057/s41599-022-01131-6

Brooks, B. D., Morrow, J. E., & Gray, W. F. (1968). Reduction of autistic gaze aversion by reinforcement of visual attention responses. *The Journal of Special Education, 2*(3), 307–309. https://doi.org/10.1177/002246696800200308

Bullen, J. C., Zajic, M. C., McIntyre, N., Solari, E., & Mundy, P. (2022). Patterns of math and reading achievement in children and adolescents with autism spectrum disorder. *Research in Autism Spectrum Disorders, 92*, 101933. https://doi.org/10.1016/j.rasd.2022.101933

Bullier, J. (2001). Integrated model of visual processing. *Brain Research Reviews, 36*(2–3), 96–107. https://doi.org/10.1016/S0165-0173(01)00085-6

Campana, F., Rebollo, I., Urai, A., Wyart, V., & Tallon-Baudry, C. (2016). Conscious vision proceeds from global to local content in goal-directed tasks and spontaneous vision. *The Journal of Neuroscience, 36*(19), 5200–5213. https://doi.org/10.1523/JNEUROSCI.3619-15.2016

Cantiani, C., Choudhury, N. A., Yu, Y. H., Shafer, V. L., Schwartz, R. G., & Benasich, A. A. (2016). From sensory perception to lexical-semantic processing: An ERP study in non-verbal children with autism. *PLoS ONE, 11*(8). https://doi.org/10.1371/journal.pone.0161637

Chawarska, K., & Shic, F. (2009). Looking but not seeing: atypical visual scanning and recognition of faces in 2 and 4-Year-old children with autism spectrum disorder. *Journal of Autism and Developmental Disorders, 39*(12), 1663–1672. https://doi.org/10.1007/s10803-009-0803-7

Chen, H., Liu, K., Zhang, B., Zhang, J., Xue, X., Lin, Y., Zou, D., Chen, M., Kong, Y., Wen, G., Yan, J., & Deng, Y. (2019). More optimal but less regulated dorsal and ventral visual networks in patients with major depressive disorder. *Journal of Psychiatric Research, 110*, 172–178. https://doi.org/10.1016/j.jpsychires.2019.01.005

Cibrian, F. L., Johnson, J., Sean, V., Pass, H., & Boyd, L. (2020). Combining Eye Tracking and Verbal Response to Understand the Impact of a Global Filter. In *Extended Abstracts of the 2020 CHI Conference on Human Factors in Computing Systems* (pp. 1–6). https://doi.org/10.1145/3334480.3382897

Cohen, E., & Kalanthroff, E. (2019). Visuospatial processing bias in ADHD: A potential artifact in the Wechsler Adult Intelligence Scale and the Rorschach Inkblots Test. *Psychological assessment, 31*(5), 699

Conway, C. M., & Christiansen, M. H. (2005). Modality-constrained statistical learning of tactile, visual, and auditory sequences. *Journal of Experimental Psychology: Learning, Memory, and Cognition, 31*, 24–39. https://doi.org/10.1037/0278-7393.31.1.24

Courchesne, E., & Pierce, K. (2005). Why the frontal cortex in autism might be talking only to itself: Local over-connectivity but long-distance disconnection. *Current Opinion in Neurobiology, 15*(2), 225–230. https://doi.org/10.1016/j.conb.2005.03.001

Dada, S., Flores, C., Bastable, K., & Schlosser, R. W. (2020). The effects of augmentative and alternative communication interventions on the receptive language skills of children with developmental disabilities: A scoping review. *International Journal of Speech-Language Pathology, 23*(3), 247–257. https://doi.org/10.1080/17549507.2020.1797165

Davidoff, J., Fonteneau, E., & Fagot, J. (2008). Local and global processing: Observations from a remote culture. *Cognition, 108*(3), 702–709. https://doi.org/10.1016/j.cognition.2008.06.004

de Jong, M. C., van ENGELAND, H., & Kemner, C. (2008). Attentional Effects of Gaze Shifts Are Influenced by Emotion and Spatial Frequency, but Not in Autism. *Journal of the American Academy of Child & Adolescent Psychiatry, 47*(4), 443–454. https://doi.org/10.1097/CHI.0b013e31816429a6

de Fockert, J. W., & Cooper, A. (2014). Higher levels of depression are associated with reduced global bias in visual processing. *Cognition and Emotion, 28*(3), 541–549. https://doi.org/10.1080/02699931.2013.839939

Deruelle, C., Rondan, C., Gepner, B., & Tardif, C. (2004). Spatial frequency and face processing in children with autism and asperger syndrome. *Journal of Autism and Developmental Disorders, 34*(2), 199–210. https://doi.org/10.1023/B:JADD.0000022610.09668.4c

Ellemberg, D., Lewis, T. L., Hong Liu, C., & Maurer, D. (1999). Development of spatial and temporal vision during childhood. *Vision Research, 39*(14), 2325–2333. https://doi.org/10.1016/S0042-6989(98)00280-6

Fink, G. R., Halligan, P. W., Marshall, J. C., Frith, C. D., Frackowiak, R. S., & Dolan, R. J. (1997). Neural mechanisms involved in the processing of global and local aspects of hierarchically organized visual stimuli. *Brain, 120*(10), 1779–1791. https://doi.org/10.1093/brain/120.10.1779

Foxton, J. M., Talcott, J. B., Witton, C., Brace, H., McIntyre, F., & Griffiths, T. D. (2003). Reading skills are related to global, but not local, acoustic pattern perception. *Nature Neuroscience, 6*, 343–344.

Franceschini, S., Bertoni, S., Gianesini, T., Gori, S., & Facoetti, A. (2017). A different vision of dyslexia: Local precedence on global perception. *Scientific Reports, 7*(1), Article 1. https://doi.org/10.1038/s41598-017-17626-1

Ganz, J. B., Hong, E. R., Goodwyn, F., Kite, E., & Gilliland, W. (2015). Impact of PECS tablet computer app on receptive identification of pictures given a verbal stimulus. *Developmental Neurorehabilitation, 18*(2), 82–87. https://doi.org/10.3109/17518423.2013.821539

Gargaro, B. A., May, T., Tonge, B. J., Sheppard, D. M., Bradshaw, J. L., & Rinehart, N. J. (2018). Attentional mechanisms in autism, ADHD, and autism-ADHD using a local-global paradigm. *Journal of Attention Disorders, 22*(14), 1320–1332. https://doi.org/10.1177/1087054715603197

Gernsbacher, M. A., & Pripas-Kapit, S. R. (2012). Who's missing the point? A commentary on claims that autistic persons have a specific deficit in figurative language comprehension. *Metaphor and Symbol, 27*(1), 93–105

Glenberg, A. M., & Kaschak, M. P. (2002). Grounding language in action. *Psychonomic Bulletin & Review, 9*(3), 558–565. https://doi.org/10.3758/BF03196313

Goldstein-Marcusohn, Y., Goldfarb, L., & Shany, M. (2020). Global and Local Visual Processing in Rate/Accuracy Subtypes of Dyslexia. *Frontiers in Psychology, 11*. https://www.frontiersin.org/article/https://doi.org/10.3389/fpsyg.2020.00828

Graham, L. (2008). Gestalt theory in interactive media design. *Journal of Humanitites and Social Science, 2*(1)

Grinter, E. J., Maybery, M. T., & Badcock, D. R. (2010). Vision in developmental disorders: Is there a dorsal stream deficit? *Brain Research Bulletin, 82*(3), 147–160. https://doi.org/10.1016/j.brainr esbull.2010.02.016

Gross, T. F. (2005). Global-local precedence in the perception of facial age and emotional expression by children with autism and other developmental disabilities. *Journal of Autism and Developmental Disorders, 35*(6), 773. https://doi.org/10.1007/s10803-005-0023-8

Guy, J., Mottron, L., Berthiaume, C., & Bertone, A. (2016). A developmental perspective of global and local visual perception in autism spectrum disorder. *Journal of Autism and Developmental Disorders.* https://doi.org/10.1007/s10803-016-2834-1

Han, S., & Humphreys, G. W. (1999). Interactions between perceptual organization based on Gestalt laws and those based on hierarchical processing. *Perception & Psychophysics, 61*(7), 1287–1298. https://doi.org/10.3758/BF03206180

Hayward, D. A., Fenerci, C., & Ristic, J. (2018). An investigation of global-local processing bias in a large sample of typical individuals varying in autism traits. *Consciousness and Cognition, 65*, 271–279. https://doi.org/10.1016/j.concog.2018.09.002

Helenius, P., Laasonen, M., Hokkanen, L., Paetau, R., & Niemivirta, M. (2011). Impaired engagement of the ventral attentional pathway in ADHD. *Neuropsychologia, 49*(7), 1889–1896. https://doi.org/10.1016/j.neuropsychologia.2011.03.014

Hill, T. L., Varela, R. E., Kamps, J. L., & Niditch, L. A. (2014). Local processing and social skills in children with Autism Spectrum Disorders: The role of anxiety and cognitive functioning. *Research in Autism Spectrum Disorders, 8*(9), 1243–1251. https://doi.org/10.1016/j.rasd.2014.06.005

Hiniker, A., Daniels, J. W., & Williamson, H. (2013). Go go games: Therapeutic video games for children with autism spectrum disorders. In *Proceedings of the 12th International Conference on Interaction Design and Children* (pp. 463–466). https://doi.org/10.1145/2485760.2485808

Huang, X., Shen, C., Boix, X., & Zhao, Q. (2015). SALICON: reducing the semantic gap in saliency prediction by adapting deep neural networks. *IEEE International Conference on Computer Vision (ICCV), 2015*, 262–270. https://doi.org/10.1109/ICCV.2015.38

Hübner, R. (1997). The effect of spatial frequency on global precedence and hemispheric differences. *Perception & Psychophysics, 59*(2), 187–201.

Hughes, H. C., Fendrich, R., & Reuter-Lorenz, P. A. (1990). Global versus local processing in the absence of low spatial frequencies. *Journal of Cognitive Neuroscience, 2*(3), 272–282. https://doi.org/10.1162/jocn.1990.2.3.272

Hughes, H. C., Nozawa, G., & Kitterle, F. (1996). Global precedence, spatial frequency channels, and the statistics of natural images. *Journal of Cognitive Neuroscience, 8*(3), 197–230. https://doi.org/10.1162/jocn.1996.8.3.197

Imbir, K. K. (2019). Does reading words differing in arousal load influence local vs. Global scope of perception? *Roczniki Psychologiczne, 22*(3), 277–297. https://doi.org/10.18290/rpsych.2019.22.3-5

Ito, J., Yamane, Y., Suzuki, M., Maldonado, P., Fujita, I., Tamura, H., & Grün, S. (2017). Switch from ambient to focal processing mode explains the dynamics of free viewing eye movements. *Scientific Reports, 7*(1), Article 1. https://doi.org/10.1038/s41598-017-01076-w

Jiang, M., Huang, S., Duan, J., & Zhao, Q. (2015). SALICON: Saliency in context. *IEEE Conference on Computer Vision and Pattern Recognition (CVPR), 2015*, 1072–1080. https://doi.org/10.1109/CVPR.2015.7298710

John, G. (1995). *Arne & Theo Engell-Nielsen.* Present and future state. University of Copenhagen.

Jolliffe, T., & Baron-Cohen, S. (1999). A test of central coherence theory: linguistic processing in high-functioning adults with autism or Asperger syndrome: is local coherence impaired?. *Cognition, 71*(2), 149–185

Jolliffe, T., & Baron-Cohen, S. (2000). Linguistic processing in high-functioning adults with autism or Asperger's syndrome. Is global coherence impaired?. *Psychological medicine, 30*(5), 1169–1187

Kaliukhovich, D. A., Manyakov, N. V., Bangerter, A., Ness, S., Skalkin, A., Boice, M., Goodwin, M. S., Dawson, G., Hendren, R., Leventhal, B., Shic, F., & Pandina, G. (2021). Visual preference for biological motion in children and adults with autism spectrum disorder: an eye-tracking study. *Journal of Autism and Developmental Disorders, 51*(7), 2369–2380. https://doi.org/10.1007/s10803-020-04707-w

Kamio, Y., Robins, D., Kelley, E., Swainson, B., & Fein, D. (2007). Atypical lexical/semantic processing in high-functioning autism spectrum disorders without early language delay. *Journal of Autism and Developmental Disorders, 37*(6), 1116–1122. https://doi.org/10.1007/s10803-006-0254-3

Katagiri, M., Kasai, T., Kamio, Y., & Murohashi, H. (2013). Individuals with Asperger's disorder exhibit difficulty in switching attention from a local level to a global level. *Journal of Autism and Developmental Disorders, 43*(2), 395–403. https://doi.org/10.1007/s10803-012-1578-9

Kihara, K., & Takeda, Y. (2019). The role of low-spatial frequency components in the processing of deceptive faces: A study using artificial face models. *Frontiers in Psychology, 10*, 1468. https://doi.org/10.3389/fpsyg.2019.01468

Koh, H. C., Milne, E., & Dobkins, K. (2010). Spatial contrast sensitivity in adolescents with autism spectrum disorders. *Journal of Autism and Developmental Disorders, 40*(8), 978–987. https://doi.org/10.1007/s10803-010-0953-7

Koldewyn, K., Jiang, Y., Weigelt, S., & Kanwisher, N. (2013). Global/local processing in autism: not a disability, but a disinclination. *Journal of Autism and Developmental Disorders, 43*(10), 2329–2340. https://doi.org/10.1007/s10803-013-1777-z

König, S. D., & Buffalo, E. A. (2014). A nonparametric method for detecting fixations and saccades using cluster analysis: Removing the need for arbitrary thresholds. *Journal of Neuroscience Methods, 227*, 121–131. https://doi.org/10.1016/j.jneumeth.2014.01.032

Lamb, M. R., & Robertson, L. C. (1990). The effect of visual angle on global and local reaction times depends on the set of visual angles presented. *Perception & Psychophysics, 47*(5), 489–496. https://doi.org/10.3758/BF03208182

Lamb, M. R., & Yund, E. W. (1996). Spatial frequency and attention: Effects of level-, target-, and location-repetition on the processing of global and local forms. *Perception & Psychophysics, 58*(3), 363–373. https://doi.org/10.3758/BF03206812

Lee, I.-J., Chen, C.-H., & Lin, L.-Y. (2016). Applied Cliplets-based half-dynamic videos as intervention learning materials to attract the attention of adolescents with autism spectrum disorder to improve their perceptions and judgments of the facial expressions and emotions of others. *Springerplus, 5*(1), 1211. https://doi.org/10.1186/s40064-016-2884-z

Liechty, J., Pieters, R., & Wedel, M. (2003). Global and local covert visual attention: Evidence from a Bayesian hidden Markov model. *Psychometrika, 68*(4), 519–541. https://doi.org/10.1007/BF02295608

Light, J., Wilkinson, K. M., Thiessen, A., Beukelman, D. R., & Fager, S. K. (2019). Designing effective AAC displays for individuals with developmental or acquired disabilities: State of the science and future research directions. *Augmentative and Alternative Communication, 35*(1), 42–55.

Lovaas, O. I., Koegel, R. L., & Schreibman, L. (1979). Stimulus overselectivity in autism: A review of research. *Psychological Bulletin, 86*, 1236–1254. https://doi.org/10.1037/0033-2909.86.6.1236

Lovaas, O. I., Schreibman, L., Koegel, R., & Rehm, R. (1971). Selective responding by autistic children to multiple sensory input. *Journal of Abnormal Psychology, 77*, 211–222. https://doi.org/10.1037/h0031015

Lu, Y., & Guo, H. (1999). Background removal in image indexing and retrieval. In *Proceedings 10th International Conference on Image Analysis and Processing* (pp. 933–938). https://doi.org/10.1109/ICIAP.1999.797715

McIntosh, R. D., & Schenk, T. (2009). Two visual streams for perception and action: Current trends. *Neuropsychologia, 47*(6), 1391–1396. https://doi.org/10.1016/j.neuropsychologia.2009.02.009

McKone, E., Aimola Davies, A., Fernando, D., Aalders, R., Leung, H., Wickramariyaratne, T., & Platow, M. J. (2010). Asia has the global advantage: Race and visual attention. *Vision Research, 50*(16), 1540–1549. https://doi.org/10.1016/j.visres.2010.05.010

Mody, R. (2022). Implications for Global and Local Visual Processing in Individuals with Learning Disabilities. *Psychology Student Papers and Posters.* https://digitalcommons.chapman.edu/psychology_student_work/1

Mottron, L., Dawson, M., Soulières, I., Hubert, B., & Burack, J. (2006). Enhanced perceptual functioning in autism: An update, and eight principles of autistic perception. *Journal of Autism and Developmental Disorders, 36*(1), 27–43. https://doi.org/10.1007/s10803-005-0040-7

Navon, D. (1969). Forest before trees: The precedence of global features in visual perception. *Perception and Psychophysics, 5*, 197–200.

Navon, D. (1977). Forest before trees: The precedence of global features in visual perception. *Cognitive Psychology, 9*(3), 353–383. https://doi.org/10.1016/0010-0285(77)90012-3

Navon, D. (1981). The forest revisited: More on global precedence. *Psychological Research Psychologische Forschung, 43*(1), 1–32. https://doi.org/10.1007/BF00309635

Nayar, K., Voyles, A. C., Kiorpes, L., & Di Martino, A. (2017). Global and local visual processing in autism: An objective assessment approach. *Autism Research, 10*(8), 1392–1404

Norman, J. (2002). Two visual systems and two theories of perception: An attempt to reconcile the constructivist and ecological approaches. *Behavioral and Brain Sciences, 25*(1), 73–96. https://doi.org/10.1017/S0140525X0200002X

O'Bryan, R. A., Brenner, C. A., Hetrick, W. P., & O'Donnell, B. F. (2014). Disturbances of visual motion perception in bipolar disorder. *Bipolar Disorders, 16*(4), 354–365. https://doi.org/10.1111/bdi.12173

O'Neill, T., Wilkinson, K. M., & Light, J. (2019). Preliminary investigation of visual attention to complex AAC visual scene displays in individuals with and without developmental disabilities. *Augmentative and Alternative Communication, 35*(3), 240–250. https://doi.org/10.1080/07434618.2019.1635643

Oliva, A., & Torralba, A. (2002). Scene-Centered Description from Spatial Envelope Properties. In H. H. Bülthoff, C. Wallraven, S.-W. Lee, & T. A. Poggio (Eds.), *Biologically Motivated Computer Vision* (pp. 263–272). Springer. https://doi.org/10.1007/3-540-36181-2_26

Oliva, A., & Schyns, P. G. (1997). Coarse blobs or fine edges? Evidence that information diagnosticity changes the perception of complex visual stimuli. *Cognitive Psychology, 34*(1), 72–107. https://doi.org/10.1006/cogp.1997.0667

Pitcher, D., & Ungerleider, L. G. (2021). Evidence for a third visual pathway specialized for social perception. *Trends in Cognitive Sciences, 25*(2), 100–110. https://doi.org/10.1016/j.tics.2020.11.006

Ploog, B. O. (2010). Stimulus overselectivity four decades later: A review of the literature and its implications for current research in autism spectrum disorder. *Journal of Autism and Developmental Disorders, 40*(11), 1332–1349. https://doi.org/10.1007/s10803-010-0990-2

Previc, F. H. (1990). Functional specialization in the lower and upper visual fields in humans: Its ecological origins and neurophysiological implications. *Behavioral and Brain Sciences, 13*(3), 519–542. https://doi.org/10.1017/S0140525X00080018

Rayner, K. (1998). Eye movements in reading and information processing: 20 years of research. *Psychological Bulletin, 124*, 372–422. https://doi.org/10.1037/0033-2909.124.3.372

Rinehart, N. J., Bradshaw, J. L., Moss, S. A., Brereton, A. V., & Tonge, B. J. (2000a). Atypical interference of local detail on global processing in high-functioning Autism and Asperger's disorder. *The Journal of Child Psychology and Psychiatry and Allied Disciplines, 41*(6), 769–778.

Rinehart, N. J., Bradshaw, J. L., Moss, S. A., Brereton, A. V., & Tonge, B. J. (2000b). Atypical interference of local detail on global processing in high-functioning Autism and Asperger's disorder. *Journal of Child Psychology and Psychiatry, 41*(6), 769–778. https://doi.org/10.1111/1469-7610.00664

Robertson, C. E., & Baron-Cohen, S. (2017). Sensory perception in autism. *Nature Reviews Neuroscience, 18*(11), 671–684. https://doi.org/10.1038/nrn.2017.112

Romski, M., Sevcik, R. A., Barton-Hulsey, A., & Whitmore, A. S. (2015). Early intervention and AAC: What a difference 30 years makes. *Augmentative and Alternative Communication, 31*(3), 181–202. https://doi.org/10.3109/07434618.2015.1064163

Rose, V., Paynter, J., Vivanti, G., Keen, D., & Trembath, D. (2020). Predictors of expressive language change for children with autism spectrum disorder receiving AAC-infused comprehensive intervention. *Journal of Autism and Developmental Disorders, 50*(1), 278–291. https://doi.org/10.1007/s10803-019-04251-2

Salvucci, D. D., & Goldberg, J. H. (2000). Identifying fixations and saccades in eye-tracking protocols. In *Proceedings of the 2000 Symposium on Eye Tracking Research & Applications* (pp. 71–78). https://doi.org/10.1145/355017.355028

Scailquin, J.-C. (2000). The fate of global precedence with age. *Experimental Aging Research, 26*(4), 285–314.

Schneps, M. H., Brockmole, J. R., Sonnert, G., & Pomplun, M. (2012). History of reading struggles linked to enhanced learning in low spatial frequency scenes. *PLoS One, 7*(4), e35724

Sean, V., Cibrian, F. L., Johnson, J., Pass, H., & Boyd, L. (2019). Poster: Toward digital image processing and eye tracking to promote visual attention for people with autism. *Ubicomp.* Ubicomp, London.

Sennott, S., & Bowker, A. (2009). Autism, AAC, and Proloquo2Go. *Perspectives on Augmentative and Alternative Communication, 18*, 137–145. https://doi.org/10.1044/aac18.4.137

Shulman, G. L., Sullivan, M. A., Gish, K., & Sakoda, W. J. (1986). The role of spatial-frequency channels in the perception of local and global structure. *Perception, 15*(3), 259–273. https://doi.org/10.1068/p150259

Shulman, G. L., & Wilson, J. (1987). Spatial Frequency and Selective Attention to Local and Global Information. *Perception, 16*(1), 89–101. https://doi.org/10.1068/p160089

Silvestre, D., Guy, J., Hanck, J., Cornish, K., & Bertone, A. (2020). Different luminance- and texture-defined contrast sensitivity profiles for school-aged children. *Scientific Reports, 10*(1), Article 1. https://doi.org/10.1038/s41598-020-69802-5

Song, Y., & Hakoda, Y. (2015). Lack of global precedence and global-to-local interference without local processing deficit: A robust finding in children with attention-deficit/hyperactivity disorder under different visual angles of the Navon task. *Neuropsychology, 29*(6), 888–894. https://doi.org/10.1037/neu0000213

Srikantharajah, J., & Ellard, C. (2022). How central and peripheral vision influence focal and ambient processing during scene viewing. *Journal of Vision, 22*(12), 4. https://doi.org/10.1167/jov.22.12.4

Staudinger, M. R., Fink, G. R., Mackay, C. E., & Lux, S. (2011). Gestalt perception and the decline of global precedence in older subjects. *Cortex, 47*(7), 854–862.

Stevenson, R. (n.d.). The impact of multisensory integration deficits on speech perception in children with autism spectrum disorders. *Frontiers in Psychology.* Retrieved March 23, 2020, from https://www.academia.edu/11058070/The_impact_of_multisensory_integration_deficits_on_speech_perception_in_children_with_autism_spectrum_disorders

Townsend, J., Harris, N. S., & Courchesne, E. (1996). Visual attention abnormalities in autism: Delayed orienting to location. *Journal of the International Neuropsychological Society, 2*(6), 541–550. https://doi.org/10.1017/S1355617700001715

Tyler, S. K., & Tucker, D. M. (1982). Anxiety and perceptual structure: Individual differences in neuropsychological function. *Journal of Abnormal Psychology, 91*, 210–220. https://doi.org/10.1037/0021-843X.91.3.210

Van Dam, W., Rueschemeyer, S.-A., Lindemann, O., & Bekkering, H. (2010). Context Effects in Embodied Lexical-Semantic Processing. *Frontiers in Psychology, 1*. https://www.frontiersin.org/articles/ https://doi.org/10.3389/fpsyg.2010.00150

Vision, N. R. C. (US) C. on. (1985). *TWO MODES OF VISUAL PROCESSING*. National Academies Press (US). https://www.ncbi.nlm.nih.gov/books/NBK219039/

Von Károlyi, C., Winner, E., Gray, W., & Sherman, G. F. (2003). Dyslexia linked to talent: Global visual-spatial ability. *Brain and language, 85*(3), 427–431

Wang, L., Mottron, L., Peng, D., Berthiaume, C., & Dawson, M. (2007). Local bias and local-to-global interference without global deficit: A robust finding in autism under various conditions of attention, exposure time, and visual angle. *Cognitive Neuropsychology, 24*(5), 550–574. https://doi.org/10.1080/13546800701417096

Wang, S., Jiang, M., Duchesne, X. M., Laugeson, E. A., Kennedy, D. P., Adolphs, R., & Zhao, Q. (2015). Atypical visual saliency in autism spectrum disorder quantified through model-based eye tracking. *Neuron, 88*(3), 604–616. https://doi.org/10.1016/j.neuron.2015.09.042

Wilkinson, K. M., & Jagaroo, V. (2004). Contributions of principles of visual cognitive science to AAC system display design. *Augmentative and Alternative Communication, 20*(3), 123–136. https://doi.org/10.1080/07434610410001699717

Wilkinson, K. M., & Madel, M. (2019). Eye tracking measures reveal how changes in the design of displays for augmentative and alternative communication influence visual search in individuals with Down syndrome or autism spectrum disorder. *American journal of speech-language pathology, 28*(4), 1649–1658

Wilkinson K. M. & Light J. (2011). Preliminary investigation of visual attention to human figures in photographs: Potential considerations for the design of aided AAC visual scene displays. *Journal of Speech, Language, and Hearing Research, 54*(6), 1644–1657. https://doi.org/10.1044/1092-4388(2011/10-0098)

Wilkinson, K. M., & Light, J. (2014). Preliminary study of gaze toward humans in photographs by individuals with autism, Down syndrome, or other intellectual disabilities: Implications for design of visual scene displays. *Augmentative and Alternative Communication, 30*(2), 130–146. https://doi.org/10.3109/07434618.2014.904434

Wong, W.-W., Rangaprakash, D., Diaz-Fong, J. P., Rotstein, N. M., Hellemann, G. S., & Feusner, J. D. (2022). Neural and behavioral effects of modification of visual attention in body dysmorphic disorder. *Translational Psychiatry, 12*(1), Article 1. https://doi.org/10.1038/s41398-022-02099-2

Xu, J., Jiang, M., Wang, S., Kankanhalli, M. S., & Zhao, Q. (2014). Predicting human gaze beyond pixels. *Journal of Vision, 14*(1), 28–28. https://doi.org/10.1167/14.1.28

Yovel, I., Revelle, W., & Mineka, S. (2005). Who sees trees before forest? The obsessive-compulsive style of visual attention. *Psychological Science, 16*(2), 123–129. https://doi.org/10.1111/j.0956-7976.2005.00792.x

From Sensory Perception to Realtime NonVerbal Communication

6

Nonverbal Communication in Autism

Nonverbal communication includes body language such as hand movements and whole body gestures, touch, time management, proximity, tone of voice, (i.e., pitch, pace, pause, frequency, volume) and speaking duration between partners, eye contact, facial expression (i.e., awareness of one's own expression and reading facial expressions of others), manners (i.e., saying "please" and "thank you"), reading the climate of a crowd, paraphrasing back to the speaker to express empathy and listening. Nonverbal communication is often considered hidden in autism as it is often conveyed via nonverbal augmentations to verbal behavior.

This hidden language dictates much of society's rules of engagement and clinicians have attempted to make this curriculum visible to autistic people through a variety of manuals such as (L. Boyd et al., 2013; Myles, 2001; Winner & Crooke, 2021). To understand how a person can display discrepancies between understanding words and not understanding nonverbal communication, one needs to consider the different processing paths for each type of information. Nonverbal communication is predominantly made up of actions (body language) and non linguistic features of spoken language such as the emotional tone of one's voice. This aspect of communication is processed through the social perception track (Belin et al., 2004).

As previously described in Chap. 1, often higher level skills on the pyramid of learning assume that lower processing skills are intact or compensate for weakness within the therapeutic environment when they develop interventions. For example, a therapist may draw a client's attention toward a social stimuli (.i.e., point and say look at this picture of a man) to then discuss it in more detail, this prompting toward social stimuli may not be embedded in the technology itself as it has been the tacit behavior of the therapist. To address when lower level skills are missing, a clinician, teacher, and caregiver intuitively

© The Author(s), under exclusive license to Springer Nature Switzerland AG 2024   85
L. Boyd, *The Sensory Accommodation Framework for Technology*, Synthesis Lectures on Technology and Health, https://doi.org/10.1007/978-3-031-48843-6_6

adapt their behavior to accommodate the visible manifestation of the sensory sensitivity. This acquiescing behavior may not be reported to researchers when they make new technologies to augment social skill therapies as it is tacit, thus making it difficult to capture prerequisite requirements of a technology system. In other words, there is hidden labor of common social skills training programs for autistic people involving the therapist engineering the physical and emotional environment for the teaching session to support the strategies employed in a session. Hidden in this context is the accommodations to compensate for sensory sensitivity. However, increasing eye contact has not generally been achieved long term through therapeutic interventions. The awareness of the connection between the perceiving the environment and responding in an expected fashion has been long held in clinical filed as evidence by pioneering researcher stated decade ago that "The failure to orient attention toward what is typically considered important in a given situation is a fundamental problem in ASD that impairs learning and the development of social skills" (Klin et al., 2003). What is still under debate is why eye contact is diminished in autism as well as how to reduce the sensory discomfort of autistic people in real time interactions.

Part 1: Sensory Environments Supports for Nonverbal Communication

As processing a complex social context requires rapid integration of multiple sensory modalities in a dynamic context (Robertson & Baron-Cohen, 2017), skill training can never fully capture or teach the existence of that context, and also fails to provide the skills needed to operate within that context. Therefore, technology needs to target support mechanisms at other processing levels beyond skill training. Some mainstream digital strategies for these behaviors such as text messages that allow for the use of punctuation, emojis, all caps, or bold–and social rules such as message at the signature line to excuse typos to not interpret as rudeness. In digitally-mediated conversations, emojis and fonts and other symbols have been used to augment meaning to capture what social communication does or face to face conversations. For example, an explicit experiment to study the use of lexical (local, word-level) and semantic (whole meaning) emojis was conducted and revealed "that participants picked more semantic suggestions than lexical suggestions and perceived the semantic suggestions as more relevant to the message content" (Zhang et al., 2021). A variety of innovative projects have been researched to support eye contact, prosody, proximity, and emotional recognition.

These approaches target long term commitment to learning or training by the user and have limited generalizability. I realized through my early work that the social skill improvements were not due to the training as much as the mediation provided by the technological system. For example, I developed and evaluated two projects to determine if systematic training could improve processing. The following projects alter nonverbal communication that occurs in face- to-face interactions using augmented reality and virtual reality. These systems were originally designed to support training of social skills, yet the user experiences highlight the foundational role that sensory modulation played in the positive outlines, therefore, designing for sensory accommodations should be a core design feature in social technologies for autism. Additionally, ensuring that the target skill is aligned with the users' social goals is also a critical aspect of design.

Technologies for Making Eye Contact

A wearable device that a caregiver dons shows promise in detecting eye contact from a child for the purpose of monitoring eye contact as an early indicator of autism (Ye et al., 2012). This system burdens the caregiver, and it is used for surveillance rather than for therapeutic or assistive purposes. Another eyeglass system is SuperGlass which is aimed to be therapeutic for a child demonstrating poor eye contact (Washington et al., 2017). A third system was deployed on mobile phones. This system, MOSOCO (Escobedo et al., 2012), digitized several lessons from a social skills curriculum (Boyd et al., 2013) and tested its efficacy with a classroom of mixed ability elementary students. One of the skills in the sequence of starting a conversation was to look at your partner. This was measured by looking through a mobile phone at one's partner and getting verification from the phone that the skills had been met. Mixed ability elementary aged children practice these skills together at their recess, allowing for the skills training to be de-stigmatized as it was used by all.

Technologies for Prosody

Technologies that aim to support normative prosody have been explored. Prosody describes the sound of speech, the way tone and other features add meaning to the words. Prosody can be used to help people interpret the meaning of their words (e.g., the tone of voice). A tablet-based system to support speech therapists when targeting the prosody of autistic children called SpeechPrompts (Simmons et al., 2014) was found to be helpful in supporting neurotypical volume and stress patterns. SayWAT is a system built on GoogleGlass™ that provides feedback to wearers about the vocal pitch patterns of themselves and their conversational partner in their immediate environment. Pitch frequency regulation is one metric for prosody, and the fluctuation in pitch provides tonal cues as the speaker's full intent.

My first project aimed to provide feedback on the speaker's tendency to use a monotone (Boyd et al., 2016) (Fig. 6.1).

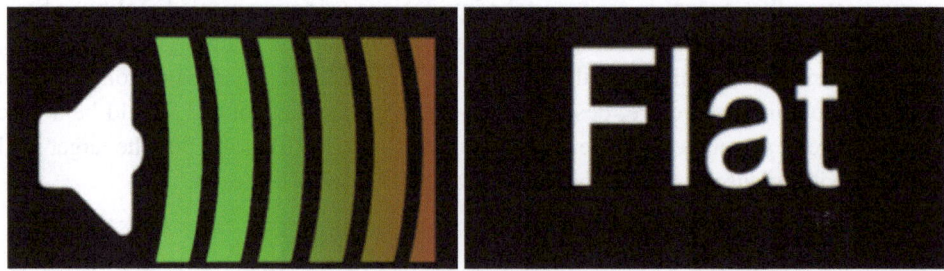

Fig. 6.1 Screenshots of sayWAT User Interfaces. Left: Speaker icon with green to red bars to indicate noise level, Right: The word "flat" to indicate a monotone voice

Prosody is also made up of the rate of speech and the use of pauses, as well as many other features. A related feature of conversational speaking is the management turn taking over time. Often it is the nonverbal aspects of one's speech that indicate if they are finished speaking or want to begin speaking. In the vrSocial project, a voice-o-meter was implemented to give mixed ability pairs persistent feedback on how much of the session they had talked. The voice-o-meter appeared at the top of the conversation partner's head in VR and was constantly updating each speaker from each end of the stats bar. Transforming the temporal activity into a visual activity allowed for the information to persist over time.

Technologies for Proximity

Proximity is the physical distance between people that is achieved and maintained as a form of communication about the relationship). I have also been explored as an assistive technology. ProCom (Boyd et al., 2017a) is an augmented reality tool aimed to support face to face communication by adding a wearable system to the physical environment. The end user wore a sensor that detected the distance of the person in front of the user and the interpersonal space (distance determined by anthropologists to be the norms by type of relationship—cultural information from (Hall, 1963) was visualized in a real-time, color-coded, two-dimensional graphic that was persistent on the mobile phone screen, see Fig. 6.2.

ProCom is an augmented reality system to visualize proximity. To visualize the nonverbal cues during face-to-face interaction, the augmented reality system consisted of a mobile phone app and a wearable sensor. The end user held a phone with a visualization of how close they were standing to an acquaintance; and they wore a sensor that detected the distance of the person in front of the user and the interpersonal space. Processing proximity requires integrating social norms with one's physical distance from others, a

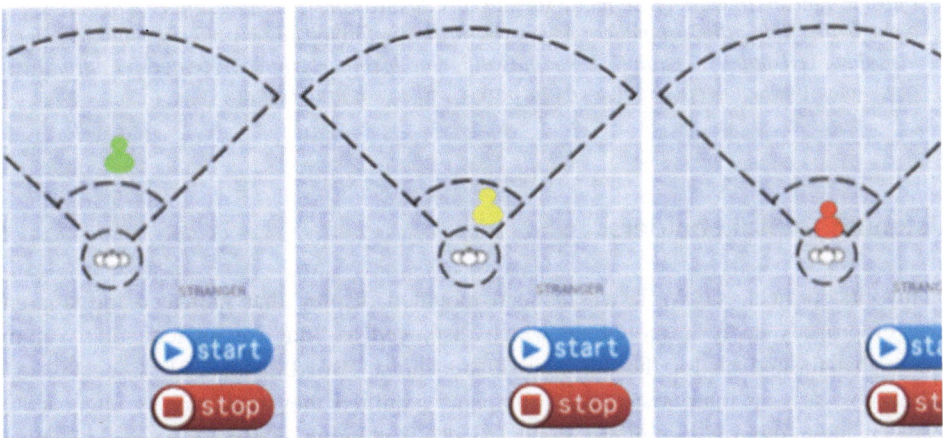

Fig. 6.2 Screenshot of ProCom interface illustrating three zones, personal zone intimate Zone and acquaintance zone. This study was calibrated for meeting someone as an acquaintance and so the green, yellow, and red people icons represent the expected, the uncomfortable and the unacceptable ranges for how close to stand to an acquaintance

task that is done in parallel with attending to the conversation. To streamline this multi-sensory processing task, proximity was visualized in real-time using color-coded zones in two-dimensional graphics.

Technologies for Emotion Recognition

Providing technical real-time support for reciprocal communication between individuals with autism and related disorders and neurotypical communicators could include selecting an emoticon that expresses emotional intent as an alternative to face-to-face nonverbal communication. Two early projects presented visuals to represent the emotion of a communication partner in real time. The first project, the Emotional Hearing Aid, uses a system to provide an interpretation of the com = conversation part's mental state and suggestions for how to react (Kaliouby & Robinson, 2005). The second project uses a system to produce "Emotion Bubbles" in realtime to help the autistic conversation partner interpret the interaction (Madsen et al., 2008). A more recent example of technology to support nonverbal communication is the augmenting of emotional recognition in Superpower glass (Washington et al., 2017). In vrSocial, I took the opposite approach by reducing the facial information using a static avatar (Boyd et al., 2018b). In vrSocial (Boyd et al., 2018b). Insights revolved around the sensory overload that was reduced in VR and makes the conversation more possible. For example, one of the mothers of two participants stated:

I love it. I mean, to work on so many social skills this way, it's an incredible way of thinking about it all. I didn't think about it that way, you're always forcing one-on-one, face-to-face. For him, there is definitely a change. It's totally different, his interactions.... He doesn't normally communicate when people come over, he barely will say hi to the adults.

Listening to Stakeholders

In my first project, sayWAT, was a head mounted display that indicated the wearer's type of prosody such as monotone which displayed as "flat" or an icon of a volume button that flashed on for the duration of loud noise (Boyd et al., 2016), see Fig. 6.1. In the post-session interviews, the participants admitted they were not as interested in feedback about themselves but did find the feedback about their partner interesting. Others in the same study went on to tell me they too had a desire to connect and make sense of the world around them. One young man indicated, "I wish I knew what people are thinking". Another stated they "would like help recognizing people, remembering names" and wanted to know topics to discuss in conversations. This insight led to designing a wearable that gave feedback about both the wearer and their interaction partner.

Reducing Multimodal Information

Participants were more interactive when using the vrSocial compared to when using Pro-Com. The mothers of the participants revealed that the sensory environment in virtual reality allows their children to feel calm and therefore more able to interact. Parents seemed to think the VR applications were better. The VR applications transformed information into an isolated visualization that could be processed as a local feature due to the low poly design that lacked details.

Parents' comments during post-session interviews provide further evidence that participants may have been calmer in the virtual reality system, versus. the augmented reality system. Parents consistently reported their children responded in a more relaxed manner in VR. I surmised that children were more comfortable due to VR allowing the designer to filter sensory input. Many mothers of the children with autism described the VR system as very visual. They acknowledged the system's primarily singular input mode. Mothers described this visual experience as comfortable for their children. A mother of twin girls whom participated in both studies stated that her reluctant daughter preferred the minimized sensory input. She described her daughter as living with vastly different sensory perceptions than those of the other people in her life:

I think they already live in their own kind of world so to them this is more normal. I think she perceives the world as, literally, a whole different place. Maybe they don't have to rely so much *on their physical senses too, maybe that overload is not as big of a problem if they are zoned in this, they don't have to feel everything*I (L. E. Boyd et al., 2018a).

VR appeared to be appealing way to reduce and control what a child with autism is experiencing. By reducing multi-sensory processing of facial expressions and body language, (see Fig. 6.3) VR can support access to new kinds of social connections (Fig. 6.4).

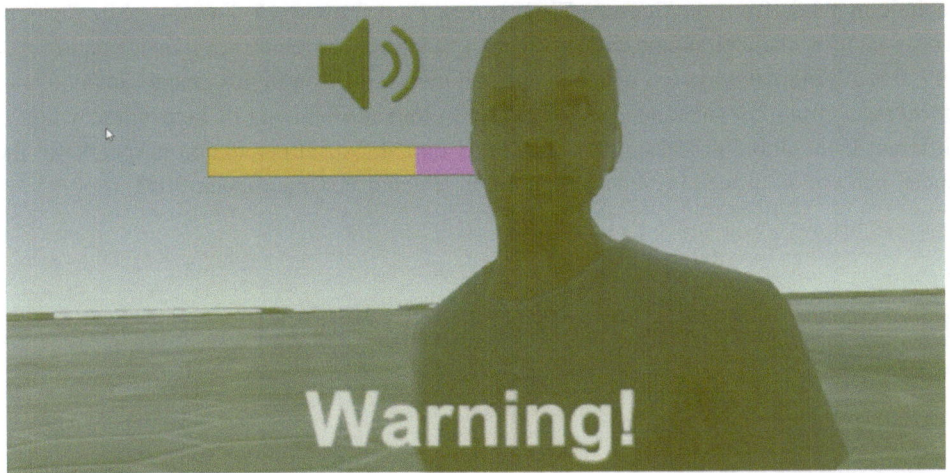

Fig. 6.3 Screenshot of the VR system with avatar of conversation partner with yellow filter and "Warning" text mid-screen and time talking bar at the top of the screen (Boyd et al., 2018b)

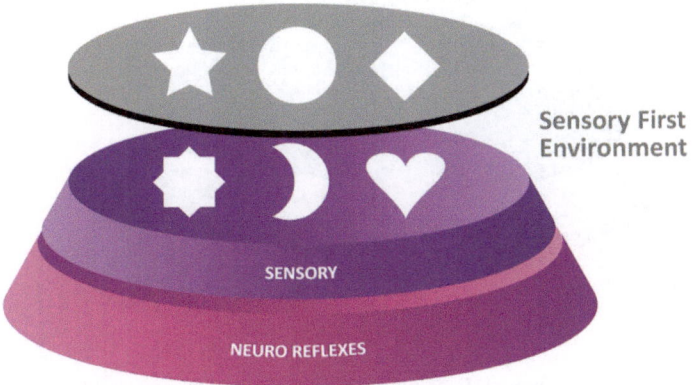

Fig. 6.4 Sensory environment-first framework model from Chap. 4

Implications for Design

People with autism may experience nonverbal communication as a hidden dimension of communication (Myles, 2001). The silent messages that are conveyed along with words are intended to clarify the meaning of the words yet can confuse people who have difficulty interpreting this form of communication. Augmenting a social interaction aims to add information about nonverbal communication (e.g., placing proximity rings on the floor or phone display). In doing so, a designer provides additional and alternative stimuli for the user to process. Details on strategies to modify the sensory environment include methods from the Sensory-Environment First framework, introduced in Chap. 4. These include channel augmentation, channel reduction, and channel transformation, see Fig. 6.5. Additional ways to engage in channel transformation in this chapter include *temporal transformation* (making persistent) and in Part 2 a blurring of faces filter which is different from global processing discussed in Chap. 4. Social perception is specific to the social perception processing track in the brain (Pitcher & Ungerleider, 2021).

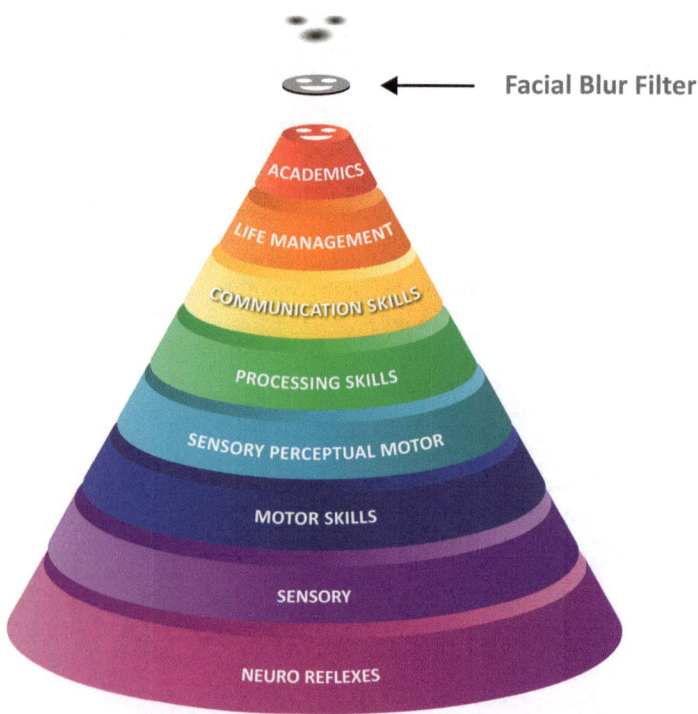

Fig. 6.5 The social comfort model. Face blurring filter applied to eyes and faces

Revisiting Channel Augmentation

Channel augmentation adds to the existing information in an environment. Specifically, the secondary information clarifies, simplifies, and highlights some aspect of the available information to be more accessible. In some cases, augmenting may be an additional burden on the user but does not distract from the social interaction. Careful design of the system interaction considers how one's gestures may impact the social interaction. For others however, managing additional information during a challenging activity may have ill effects, as mentioned previously by parents whose children participated in both my AR and VR nonverbal communication studies. Perhaps the wearer attends to the alternative information by instead of attending to the social partner. In this case, the system augments with alternative information and filters out less desirable input, therefore serving as an "involvement shield" (Humphreys, 2005).

Revisiting Channel Reduction

For people with sensory integration difficulties, much energy is directed at tolerating the ample sensory experiences rather than at learning new information efficiently. To circumvent these discomforts, reduce the sheer amount of information or strain out the "rich media"(Daft & Lengel, 1986). Rich media contains multiple sources of information to replicate the richness of face-to-face interactions. Face-to-face interactions include tone of voice, eye contact, body language and more.

Revisiting Channel Transformation

Filtering sensory information to resemble *lean media*, media with a limited amount of information (Daft & Lengel, 1986) to ease user experience. In the VR system, I transformed social information into a more accessible format via text and color coding. The text is an object that gets processed locally and globally (Goldstein-Marcusohn et al., 2020) whereas color gets processed by the local stream (Claeys et al., 2004). It stated that the user was standing "too close" to the other. If the users were violating the personal space of the other, the text read "step back". I also obscured the conversation partner from view with colored filters. Much the stimuli in the virtual environment is visual; nonverbal communication information appeared graphically. I chose graphic data visualizations (i.e., combination of symbols, icons, and text to convey a message). Although the graphics were not completely static, they were persistent in the virtual environment, creating a continual presence.

vrSocial uses visual input to convey otherwise hidden information—volume, interpersonal space, and the time one spends talking in the conversation, see Fig. 6.3. It demonstrated ways to visualize auditory, perceptual, and temporal information; however, this could be extended to all the channels. vrSocial reduced the overall sensory experiences using minimal background environment, the static body of the avatar (i.e., only whole-body movements such as floating back and forth), minimal use of color and texture, audio exclusively from the other person's headset, and no haptic feedback. Only objects or people that are part of the task at hand were included to reduce distraction while supporting attention to the conversation. By reducing the overall sensory load, users have more opportunity to interact without sensory distractions.

Part 2: Social Perceptual Processing of Eye Gaze

Researchers have recently identified the location of the "social brain" that has been part of some autism theories for some time. This third visual attention pathway is on the lateral brain surface (Pitcher & Ungerleider, 2021), whereas the global! is on the dorsal side and the location is on the ventral side. The third pathway processes visual stimuli in motion, specifically facial expressions and body movements (Pitcher & Ungerleider, 2021). Regarding the differences in the social perceptual pathway, researchers have recently concluded that eye avoidance of social content such as faces is used "to reduce amygdala-related hyperarousal among people on the autism spectrum." (Stuart et al., 2022). The social perceptual stream has also been linked to processing the perceived messages conveyed through voice, as well as the audio-visual integration of speech (Pitcher & Ungerleider, 2021).

Links between difficulties with face processing have long been reported in research on autism (Almourad & Bataineh, 2020; Boyd et al., 2016; Deruelle et al., 2004; McPartland et al., 2011; Nickl-Jockschat et al., 2015; Solomon-Harris, 2022; Speer et al., 2007; Tanaka et al., 2010). The third stream is a recent finding that "computes a range of higher sociocognitive functions based on dynamic social cues. These include facial expression recognition, eye gaze discrimination, the audiovisual integration of speech, and interpreting the actions and behaviors of other biological organisms" (Pitcher & Ungerleider, 2021). The third stream incorporates motion information and other "sensory modalities in order to support the ability to understand and interpret the actions of others" (Solomon-Harris, 2022).

Human faces and eyes in motion have been found to result in "sensory hyperresponsiveness in young autistic individuals" (Jones et al., 2018). A hyperarousal state can occur even when a person is hyposensitive in other contexts (Chen et al., 2022). Several studies have confirmed that autistic children tend to avoid the eyes when they are looking at faces (Xu & Tanaka, 2013). "Studies of eye gaze have indicated that "eye avoidance is a strategy used to reduce amygdala-related hyperarousal for people on the autism spectrum" (Stuart et al., 2022). Tanaka and coauthors designed and evaluated a face training program and found it to be effective training face processing for young autistic adults (Tanaka et al., 2010). An alternative to face processing training is accommodating sensory processing challenges by changing the social stimuli to be more comfortable and therefore accessible, see Fig. 6.5. As voices of Autistic participants confirm that viewing faces in real time conversations can result in "adverse emotional and physiological reactions, feelings of being invaded, and sensory overload while making eye contact, in addition to difficulties understanding social nuances, and difficulties receiving and sending nonverbal information" (Trevisan et al., 2017), it is imperative technology designs aim to make people feel safe.

Implications for Design: Sensory Accommodation Framework Design Principles

Implications for social communication design at the top layer of the sensory accommodation framework, after sensory input from the system has been filtered through the other three layers. What is left is now complex social information and other information that is expected to be learned. At this stage because of the dynamic nature of information and the fear associated with looking at faces and eyes it's been documented repeatedly by researchers and autistic people alike, removing the aversive stimulus is the goal here for accessing real time interactions and learning opportunities. This may require transforming all sensory input into a single channel–unisensory. This degree of flattening ensures that the information has a high likelihood of being filtered sufficiently.

Another mechanism for this level of design is to find a way to make rapidly changing information more permanent and therefore accessible for people that have a longer window of binding two or more modalities together. "Freezing the screen" to provide some sense of persistence as well as other ways to customize the time that the users are exposed to the stimuli will help with the temporal multisensory processing difficulties in autism.

Conclusion

Social skills have long been a focus of intervention for autistic people. this chapter as well as this whole book is designed to redirect attention from training social skills to the foundational sensory processing skills that impact one's ability to engage in neurotypical social behavior. Regardless, if one is motivated to participate in mainstream expectations, there are many challenges, most notably in this chapter, regarding the difficulties with social perception processing. Social skills are often described as the hidden curriculum to autistic people because they are accessories to more direct behavior like spoken language.

and they occur at the same time and are difficult to integrate so often go less noticed. Designers could support the challenges with the social perceptual pathway by making social information more explicit without burdening the user to perform a particular skill, but rather relieve them of the multisensory processing over time that's required of social interaction and provide some metadata.

Designing systems that augment nonverbal communication in a sensory modality that is a strength or preference could alleviate the burden of interpreting multiple signals at once. as it's been known that faces cause hyperarousal and some people with autism (Stuart et al., 2022), reducing this fear response at the onset could change the social opportunities for people. For many decades researchers have been aware that autistic people have a fear response to social stimuli particularly faces and eyes and yet the only interventions available are to train eye contact and somehow desensitize people to these fearful stimuli. However, an assistive technology and accessible technology would take the opposite approach and reduce or minimize the unwanted simulation and replace it with a comfortable environment. It is the goal of this Chap. 2 to reiterate that therapeutic and assistive technologies aimed at social support can be Bridge together with a consideration of the context and goal of the person if someone wants to work on learning a new skill and practicing it in a safe environment than a therapeutic technology maybe what they're looking for, if they're looking for performing out in the world, training is not the tool they are likely to employ rather a tool that makes the world accessible to them would be more appropriate for social world. in the future as technologies become increasing made up of mixed reality platforms and ubiquitous environments, the opportunity for this sort of approach will be exponential.

References

Almourad, M. B., & Bataineh, E. (2020). Visual attention toward human face recognizing for autism spectrum disorder and normal developing children: An eye tracking study. In *Proceedings of the 2020 The 6th International Conference on E-Business and Applications* (pp. 99–104). https://doi.org/10.1145/3387263.3387283

Belin, P., Fecteau, S., & Bédard, C. (2004). Thinking the voice: Neural correlates of voice perception. *Trends in Cognitive Sciences, 8*(3), 129–135. https://doi.org/10.1016/j.tics.2004.01.008

Boyd, L., McReynolds, C., & Chanin, K. (2013). *The Social Compass Curriculum.* Paul Brookes Publishing, Inc. https://products.brookespublishing.com/The-Social-Compass-Curriculum-P687.aspx

Boyd, L. E., Rangel, A., Tomimbang, H., Conejo-Toledo, A., Patel, K., Tentori, M., & Hayes, G. R. (2016). SayWAT: Augmenting face-to-face conversations for adults with autism. In *Proceedings of the 2016 CHI Conference on Human Factors in Computing Systems* (pp. 4872–4883). https://doi.org/10.1145/2858036.2858215

Boyd, L. E., Jiang, X., & Hayes, G. R. (2017). ProCom: Designing and evaluating a mobile and wearable system to support proximity awareness for people with autism. In *Proceedings of the 2017 CHI Conference on Human Factors in Computing Systems* (pp. 2865–2877). https://doi.org/10.1145/3025453.3026014

Boyd, L. E., Ringland, K. E., Faucett, H., Hiniker, A., Klein, K., Patel, K., & Hayes, G. R. (2017). Evaluating an iPad game to address overselectivity in preliterate AAC users with minimal verbal behavior. In *Proceedings of the 19th International ACM SIGACCESS Conference on Computers and Accessibility* (pp. 240–249). https://doi.org/10.1145/3132525.3132551

Boyd, L. E., Gupta, S., Vikmani, S. B., Gutierrez, C. M., Yang, J., Linstead, E., & Hayes, G. R. (2018a). vrSocial: Toward immersive therapeutic VR systems for children with autism. In *Proceedings of the 2018 CHI Conference on Human Factors in Computing Systems* (pp. 1–12). https://doi.org/10.1145/3173574.3173778

Boyd, L. E., Gupta, S., Vikmani, S. B., Gutierrez, C. M., Yang, J., Linstead, E., & Hayes, G. R. (2018b). vrSocial: Toward immersive therapeutic VR systems for children with autism. In *Proceedings of the 2018 CHI Conference on Human Factors in Computing Systems* (pp. 1–12). https://doi.org/10.1145/3173574.3173778

Chen, Y.-J., Harrop, C., Sabatos-DeVito, M., Bulluck, J., Belger, A., & Baranek, G. (2022). Brief report: Attention patterns to non-social stimuli and associations with sensory features in autistic children. *Research in Autism Spectrum Disorders, 98*, 102035. https://doi.org/10.1016/j.rasd.2022.102035

Claeys, K. G., Dupont, P., Cornette, L., Sunaert, S., Van Hecke, P., De Schutter, E., & Orban, G. A. (2004). Color discrimination involves ventral and dorsal stream visual areas. *Cerebral Cortex (New York, N.Y.: 1991), 14*(7), 803–822. https://doi.org/10.1093/cercor/bhh040

Daft, R. L., & Lengel, R. H. (1986). Organizational information requirements, media richness and structural design. *Management Science, 32*(5), 554–571.

Deruelle, C., Rondan, C., Gepner, B., & Tardif, C. (2004). Spatial frequency and face processing in children with autism and Asperger syndrome. *Journal of Autism and Developmental Disorders, 34*(2), 199–210. https://doi.org/10.1023/B:JADD.0000022610.09668.4c

Du, Y., Boyd, L., & Ibrahim, S. (2018). *From Behavioral and Communication Intervention to Interaction Design: User Perspectives from Clinicians.* 6

Escobedo, L., Nguyen, D. H., Boyd, L., Hirano, S., Rangel, A., Garcia-Rosas, D., Tentori, M., & Hayes, G. (2012). MOSOCO: A mobile assistive tool to support children with autism practicing social skills in real-life situations. In *Proceedings of the SIGCHI Conference on Human Factors in Computing Systems* (pp. 2589–2598). https://doi.org/10.1145/2207676.2208649

Goldstein-Marcusohn, Y., Goldfarb, L., & Shany, M. (2020). Global and local visual processing in rate/accuracy subtypes of dyslexia. *Frontiers in Psychology, 11*. https://www.frontiersin.org/article/https://doi.org/10.3389/fpsyg.2020.00828

Hall, E. T. (1963). A system for the notation of proxemic behavior. *American Anthropologist, 65*(5), 1003–1026.

Humphreys, L. (2005). Cellphones in public: social interactions in a wireless era. *New Media & Society, 7*(6), 810–833. https://doi.org/10.1177/1461444805058164

Kaliouby elRobinson, R. (2005). The emotional hearing aid: An assistive tool for children with Asperger syndrome. *Universal Access in the Information Society, 4*(2), 121–134. https://doi.org/10.1007/s10209-005-0119-0

Klin, A., Jones, W., Schultz, R., & Volkmar, F. (2003). The enactive mind, or from actions to cognition: Lessons from autism. *Philosophical Transactions of the Royal Society b: Biological Sciences, 358*(1430), 345–360. https://doi.org/10.1098/rstb.2002.1202

Madsen, M., el Kaliouby, R., Goodwin, M., & Picard, R. (2008). Technology for just-in-time in-situ learning of facial affect for persons diagnosed with an autism spectrum disorder. In *Proceedings of the 10th International ACM SIGACCESS Conference on Computers and Accessibility* (pp. 19–26). https://doi.org/10.1145/1414471.1414477

McPartland, J. C., Webb, S. J., Keehn, B., & Dawson, G. (2011). Patterns of visual attention to faces and objects in autism spectrum disorder. *Journal of Autism and Developmental Disorders, 41*(2), 148–157. https://doi.org/10.1007/s10803-010-1033-8

Mundy, P., Sigman, M., Ungerer, J., & Sherman, T. (1987). Nonverbal communication and play correlates of language development in autistic children. *Journal of Autism and Developmental Disorders, 17*(3), 349–364. https://doi.org/10.1007/BF01487065

Myles, B. S. (2001). Understanding the hidden curriculum: an essential social skill for children and youth with asperger syndrome. *Intervention in School and Clinic, 36*(5), 279–286. https://doi.org/10.1177/105345120103600504

Nickl-Jockschat, T., Rottschy, C., Thommes, J., Schneider, F., Laird, A. R., Fox, P. T., & Eickhoff, S. B. (2015). Neural networks related to dysfunctional face processing in autism spectrum disorder. *Brain Structure and Function, 220*(4), 2355–2371. https://doi.org/10.1007/s00429-014-0791-z

Noel, J.-P., De Niear, M. A., Lazzara, N. S., & Wallace, M. T. (2018). Uncoupling between multisensory temporal function and nonverbal turn-taking in autism spectrum disorder. *IEEE Transactions on Cognitive and Developmental Systems, 10*(4), 973–982. https://doi.org/10.1109/TCDS.2017.2778141

Pitcher, D., & Ungerleider, L. G. (2021). Evidence for a third visual pathway specialized for social perception. *Trends in Cognitive Sciences, 25*(2), 100–110. https://doi.org/10.1016/j.tics.2020.11.006

Robertson, C. E., & Baron-Cohen, S. (2017). Sensory perception in autism. *Nature Reviews Neuroscience, 18*(11), 671–684. https://doi.org/10.1038/nrn.2017.112

Simmons, E. S., Paul, R., & Shic, F. (2014). *The Use of Mobile Technology in the Treatment of Prosodic Deficits in Autism Spectrum Disorders.*

Solomon-Harris, L. M. (2022). *Atypical Lateralization of Language and Face Processing in Autism Spectrum Disorder.* https://yorkspace.library.yorku.ca/xmlui/handle/10315/39586

Speer, L. L., Cook, A. E., McMahon, W. M., & Clark, E. (2007). Face processing in children with autism: Effects of stimulus contents and type. *Autism, 11*(3), 265–277. https://doi.org/10.1177/1362361307076925

Spiel, K., Frauenberger, C., Keyes, O., & Fitzpatrick, G. (2019). Agency of autistic children in technology research: A critical literature review. *ACM Transactions on Computer-Human Interaction, 26*(6), 38:1–38:40. https://doi.org/10.1145/3344919

Stuart, N., Whitehouse, A., Palermo, R., Bothe, E., & Badcock, N. (2022). Eye gaze in autism spectrum disorder: a review of neural evidence for the eye avoidance hypothesis. *Journal of Autism and Developmental Disorders.* https://doi.org/10.1007/s10803-022-05443-z

Tanaka, J., Wolf, J., & Schultz, R. (2010). The Let's Face It! Program: The assessment and treatment of face processing deficits in children with autism spectrum disorder. *Journal of Vision - J VISION, 10*, 593–593. https://doi.org/10.1167/10.7.593

Trevisan, D. A., Roberts, N., Lin, C., & Birmingham, E. (2017). How do adults and teens with self-declared Autism Spectrum Disorder experience eye contact? A qualitative analysis of first-hand accounts. *PLoS ONE, 12*(11), e0188446. https://doi.org/10.1371/journal.pone.0188446

Washington, P., Voss, C., Kline, A., Haber, N., Daniels, J., Fazel, A., De, T., Feinstein, C., Winograd, T., & Wall, D. (2017). SuperpowerGlass: A wearable aid for the at-home therapy of children with autism. *Proceedings of the ACM on Interactive, Mobile, Wearable and Ubiquitous Technologies, 1*(3), 112:1–112:22. https://doi.org/10.1145/3130977

Winner, M. G., & Crooke, P. (2021). *You Are a Social Detective!: Explaining Social Thinking to Kids, 2nd Edition.* Think Social Publishing.

Xu, B., & Tanaka, J. (2013). *Teaching Children with Autism to Recognize Faces.* https://doi.org/10.1007/978-1-4614-4788-7_56

Ye, Z., Li, Y., Fathi, A., Han, Y., Rozga, A., Abowd, G. D., & Rehg, J. M. (2012). Detecting eye contact using wearable eye-tracking glasses. In *Proceedings of the 2012 ACM Conference on Ubiquitous Computing* (pp. 699–704). https://doi.org/10.1145/2370216.2370368

Zhang, M. "Ray," Mariakakis, A., Burke, J., & Wobbrock, J. O. (2021). A Comparative Study of Lexical and Semantic Emoji Suggestion Systems. In K. Toeppe, H. Yan, & S. K. W. Chu (Eds.), *Diversity, Divergence, Dialogue* (Vol. 12645, pp. 229–247). Springer International Publishing. https://doi.org/10.1007/978-3-030-71292-1_20

Timing is Everything: Temporal Processing and MultiSensory Integration

7

Designing Beyond a Label

This book up to this chapter has focused on autism and the many layers of processing that occur rapidly as an autistic person engages with the world. Many of these differences are experienced by the broader neurodivergent community as well. Neurodivergence refers to variation in the human experience (*Neurodiversity—NCI*, 2022). Most commonly considered to refer to, but not limited to, conditions such as autism, ADHD, and dyslexia. All three share commonalities in sensory processing differences, however they each have distinct diagnostic criteria.

Clinically, autism is a variation of the human condition that is characterized by social communication difficulties as well as repetitive or restricted behaviors or thoughts. Autism has a prevalence rate of 17% in the United States (CDC, 2023). ADHD is a condition that is characterized by inattention, hyperactivity, and impulsivity. ADHD has a prevalence rate of just under 10% in the United States (CDC, 2022). The co-occurrence of autism and ADHD is 50–70% (Hours et al., 2022). Dyslexia is characterized as slow or poor reading and spelling without a cause due to intelligence or sensory abilities (Formoso et al., 2022). Dyslexia has an estimated prevalence of 7% (Peterson & Pennington, 2012). The co-occurrence of ADHD and dyslexia is 20–40% in the United States (McGrath & Stoodley, 2019). Collectively, neurodivergence represents 15–20% of the world's population (*Neurodiversity—NCI*, 2022). Given the overlap in symptomatology, there is a need to "move from mutually exclusive diagnostic categories to behavioural profiles" (Brimo et al., 2021). As these main neurodivergence are a substantially large yet an underserved community to consider in the design of all technologies, but particularly in the design of assistive and accessible technologies.

L. Boyd, *The Sensory Accommodation Framework for Technology*, Synthesis Lectures on Technology and Health, https://doi.org/10.1007/978-3-031-48843-6_7

This chapter focuses on the common challenges across the three main conditions that can be leveraged to support neurodiverse designs. The goal being that by focusing on subsets of processing, designers can not only provide more tailored support but also move away from diagnostic labels that may confine a design to a person that does not fit any particular individual. The design of accessible technologies needs to focus on the flexibility required to meet the numerous ephemeral instantaneous processes that occur in rapidly over time.

Target Processing Types, Not a Condition

Similar atypical neurological processes exist across neurodivergence. As neurological processing occurs rapidly across the brain and is immensely complex, this chapter will only discuss a few common processes that are central to neurodivergent conditions. Understanding these core processes as sites for technology design may be more helpful than attempting to target a specific condition. Conditions are made up of multiple diagnostic criteria that may not meet any one particular person's needs, but rather convey a "persona" of the condition. Therefore, targeting the core sub processes can perhaps meet specific needs for many people, perhaps even those who do not identify as neurodivergent. For example, there are a variety of theories about the neurological cause(s) of dyslexia. As (Goldstein-Marcusohn et al., 2020) explained, some researchers have defined dyslexia as a phonological deficit (Shankweiler and Liberman, 1989) while other researchers (Wolf and Bowers, 1999) have found sub processes of phonological awareness to be unhindered. (Goldstein-Marcusohn et al., 2020) added that other researchers have identified a variety of visual attention differences in dyslexia. As our understanding of the brain continues to expand, our methods of more inclusive technology must expand too.

Below are sections for each processing domain, broken down by condition because this is how clinical research presents findings—by diagnosis. Reading across these diagnoses will provide an understanding of how neurodivergence presents across a spectrum. The goal of this Chapter is to provide insight from varied neurodivergent experiences related to multisensory integration, as well as temporal processing of static and dynamic stimuli. Both are required for processing of information to occur across the sensory to cognitive workflow.

Multisensory Integration Differences in Neurodivergence

As mentioned in Chap. 4, each sensory modality singularly can be challenging for autism, but a particular challenge is multi modal integration. Specific challenges exist in autism regarding integrating multiple inputs such as visuo-spatial, auditory-temporal, global–local processing. These challenges occur to the degree that researchers hypothesize that autistics may engage in *channel switching* **between two modalities** (Little et al., 2017) and *sensory conservation,* specifically reducing visual stimuli to reduce the overload of multisensory integration (Humphreys, 2005). In addition to single channel sensitivities described in Chap. 3, people with autism may find the ongoing integration of information received through multiple channels to be burdensome (Bogdashina, 2016; Foss-Feig et al., 2010; Noel et al., 2018; Robertson & Baron-Cohen, 2017).

Combining sensory information from visual and auditory channels is a core process and is required to comprehend language. Face to face language processing requires the integration of vocal and facial cues (Kuhl & Meltzoff, 1982). Researchers have demonstrated the difficulty synchronizing nonverbal communication with multisensory temporal processing (Noel et al., 2018). Additionally, researchers have found that autistic children have decreased benefit from multisensory stimuli when taught reading at the word-level. They needed the signal to noise ratio to extract meaning at the level of whole-word recognition" (Stevenson et al., 2017). Taken together, supporting the integration of multiple sensory channels could support access to the communication and the social world. Therefore, it is imperative that technology designs can consider strategies that offload the work of channel switching and channel conservation can be leveraged to improve delivering of information via assistive technology systems. There are opportunities at each layer of the Sensory Accommodation Framework for Technology to assist with the integration of multiple sensory streams, with specific opportunities at the bottom layer of Sensory-First Environments accommodations where the sensory stimuli can be reduced or transformed, see Fig. 7.1.

Additionally, this same level can be applied to the same multisensory integration difficulties in ADHD, that is likely to co-occur with autism. Sensory processing hypersensitivity in ADHD has been characterized as "being flooded by sensory events" and difficulty filtering out background noise (Little et al., 2017). Some researchers have found audiovisual integration to occur faster in adults with ADHD than neurotypical controls (McCracken et al., 2019). This alternative experience of processing faster than typical has been used as an explanation for distractibility as the person with ADHD seeks out other stimuli while waiting (Schulze et al., 2020). In other words, the hypothesized low thresholds to stimuli in ADHD result in a strategy that is labeled as distraction. (See Chap. 3 for more details on designing for a range in neurological thresholds and self-regulation needs).

Difficulties combining visual-spatial and auditory perception have been linked to dyslexia. Several different theories exists as to what these interaction between multisensory processes are(Goldstein-Marcusohn et al., 2020), further underscoring the need to make flexible systems that can be calibrated to each user's specific profile. Different types of reading disorders may exist because of the myriad of aspects involved in reading.

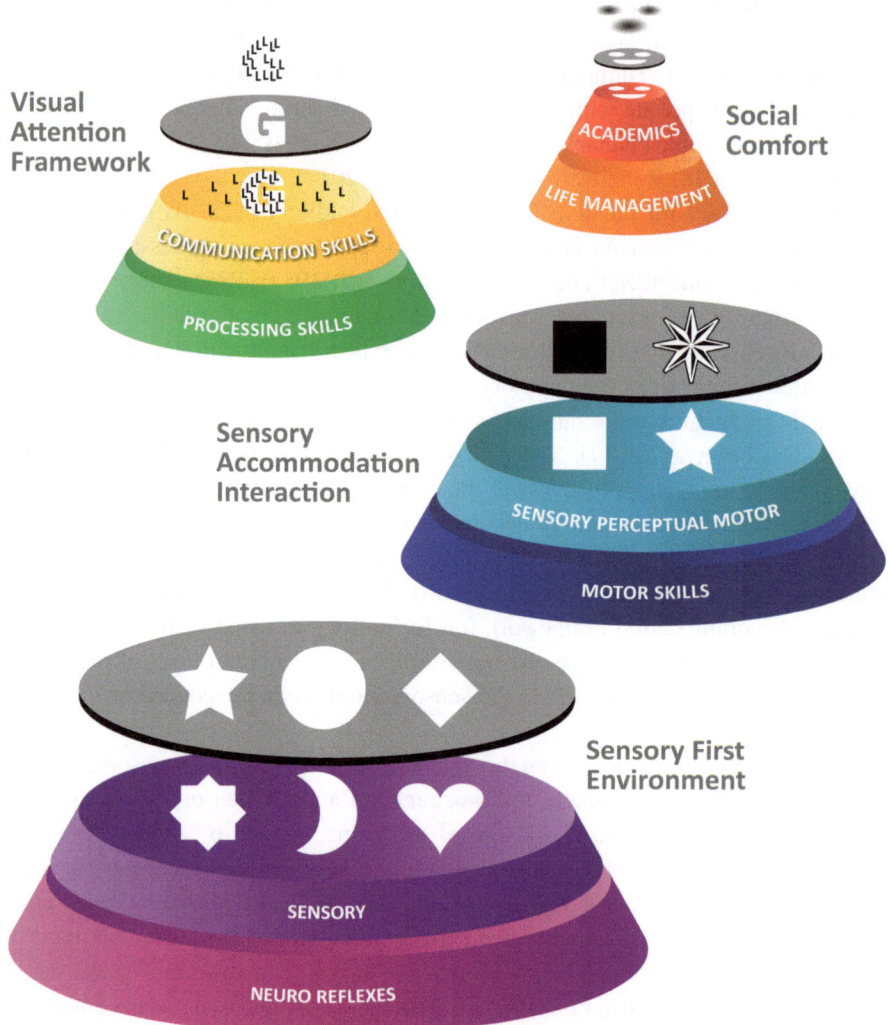

Fig. 7.1 Four layers of the sensory accommodation framework

Temporal Processing of MultiSensory Information

Temporal Processing is a key aspect of sensory processing. Neurological processing occurs instantly as well as over time. The passing of time is a process in and of itself where incoming stimulation is bound together. "Auditory temporal processing can be defined as the perception of sound or of the alteration of sound within a restricted or defined time domain" (Shinn, 2003). So too does visual, tactile, and all other sensory input continuously and simultaneously pour into the nervous system and require ongoing temporal processing. Temporal processing occurs for static and dynamic (in motion) information. Although a number of superior perceptual abilities exist among people with autism (Mottron et al., 2006), the difficulty with temporal processing of multisensory information beginning at low levels has repercussions on high level processing (Stevenson et al., 2014).

Temporal processing not only integrates sensory information from multiple sensory channels, it also separates and combines signals (Robertson & Baron-Cohen, 2017). In other words, the event timing plays a role in how, what, and when information is processed. For example, part of comprehending the multiple cues exchanged during a face-to-face conversation involves not only integrating verbal and nonverbal behavior but also noticing the duration and sequencing of each as well. For people with autism, slower temporal processing is associated with difficulties with social interaction (Robertson & Baron-Cohen, 2017). Specifically, recent studies have found that "this poor multisensory temporal acuity appears to be strongly related to the communicative challenges frequently observed" in autism (Daft & Lengel, 1986). Therefore, designing technology to support the temporal processing, multisensory processing may exemplify "value added automation" (Horvitz, 1999). Thus, designing a technology that segregates or combines multiple types of information can be advantageous because we are able to control the system's sensory load, adapting it to meet the individual's sensory processing needs.

Temporal processing further complicates sensory processing when stimuli input is continuous and begins to build up over time. Integrating unisensory, multiple sensory and hierarchical global and local information rapidly occurs over time. Audition, vision, and touch involve temporal processing (Conway & Christiansen, 2005; Kubovy, 1988).

The processing window in which different sensory modalities are bound together has been found to be larger in autism (Robertson & Baron-Cohen, 2017). The timing window is critical to determining which bits of information to put together into one event or not perceived as part of the same event (Meilleur et al., 2020), see Fig. 7.2. The larger temporal binding window results in events being perceptive as occurring simultaneously when they are not (Meilleur et al., 2020). This mis-timing may result in difficulty with high level processing such as speech recognition (Meilleur et al., 2020).

One theory of ADHD is that the temporal processing is altered such that people with ADHD have a different perception of time (Sonuga-Barke et al., 2010). However, similar to autism and dyslexia, no one theory accounts for heterogeneity in symptoms in ADHD (Sonuga-Barke et al., 2010). Similar findings of disruption integration of auditory integration over time have been found in dyslexia (Formoso et al., 2022). In dyslexia, the disrupted temporal processing has been indicated in auditory processing and audio-visual processing where the order of sounds or the order of two stimuli are not corrected (Meilleur et al., 2020). Therefore, with the abundance of temporal processing difficulties, designing for variations in sensory processing is warranted.

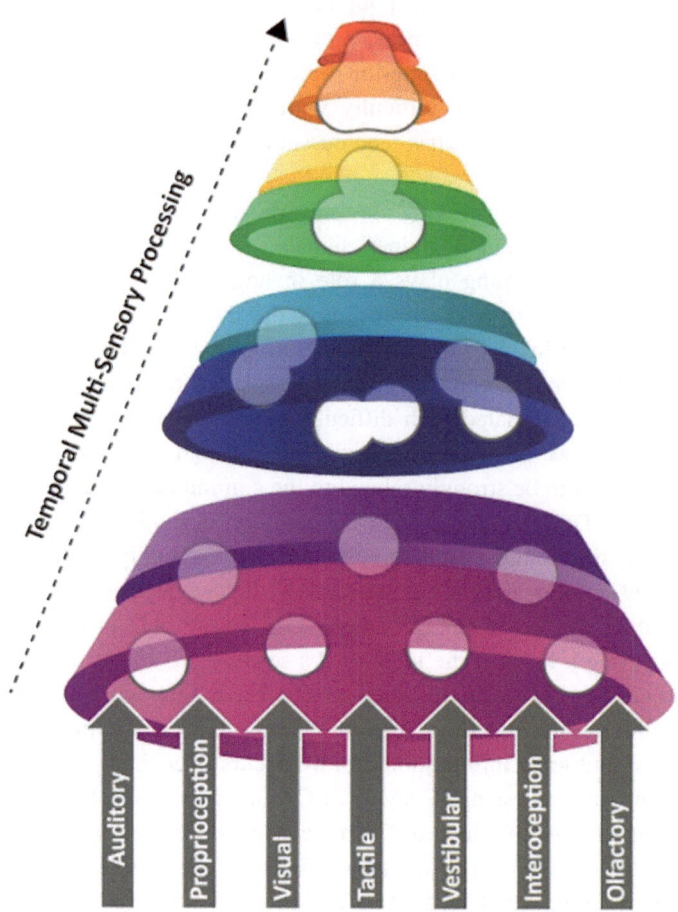

Fig. 7.2 Temporal processing layer for multisensory integration. Seven sensory modalities are shown as entering into a system and represented as circles. As these sensory modalities enter into the learning cone at the same time, they are merged together as they increasingly become more and more integrated over time, resulting in a single event or experience at the top of the cone

Some technology workarounds that change the perception modality such as with dyslexia, which has been addressed by changing the color of a screen to warm colors lead to faster reading (Rello & Bigham, 2017). These findings are supported by neuroscience that ties these findings to global track difficulties: Difficulties with processing of global information in dyslexia have been supported by addressing low level features such as the color of the background. reading text that on blue or yellow may improve progress because yellow and blue cones stimulate the global pathway at a preconscious level (Stein, 2014). The global pathway receives signals from red and green cones that are "activated by yellow light" (Stein, 2014).

Furthermore, researchers have found reduced sensitivity to low contrast stimuli processed by the global track resulted in difficulties with fixating on a letter when reading, hence the sense that the letter is moving around (Ali et al., 2021). Developers have explored bolding the letters (*Bionic Reading*, n.d.); the initial letters of a word have a mechanism to support issues with ADHD and dyslexia in terms of organizing the *temporal pattern* of reading. The mechanism is to bold the first letters of a word to anchor where to start (see website bionic-reading dot com). Additionally, systematic exploration of the shape of letter via fonts have been found impacts the complexity of low level processing) has been utilized to allow for the information to be more easily understood (Rello & Baeza-Yates, 2016).

With an understanding of dynamic multisensory integration and hierarchical processing, design decisions can be planned out systematically. Researchers have found that manipulating stimuli at the global level (e.g., Navon figures) might increase reading ability and attention (Franceschini et al., 2017).

Implication for Temporal MultiSensory Integration Design

Several strategies can be employed to support disrupted temporal processing of unisensory and multi-sensory integrations. These design features can support temporal processing at any of the layers and have been discussed by layer in previous chapters.

Flattening Stimuli to Unisensory (Autism)

To address the burden of multisensory integration, transform all input to unisensory input. The channel transformation at the sensory-environment first layer can work around the need to switch channels form one to the other (Channel switching) or ignore one channel to converse processing efforts (Channel conservation), see Fig. 7.2.

Screen Out Background Information that is a Distraction

To address distraction, screen out background stimuli (low detection threshold) is a way to support distraction. Referring to the Visual Attention layer of the Sensory Accommodation Framework, the global filter will provide the most salient information to guide visual attention of the user, although those with ADHD can get distracted, a response to regulate low sensory threshold.

Anchor Key Information (Dyslexia)

Both to support the temporal challenges and neurodiverse conditions, anchoring important stimuli can extend the processing time enough to make information comprehendible. examples of anchors that could be supportive and dyslexia are visual-spatial anchors for start points to show where to start reading as provided by the bionic reading program (*Bionic Reading*, n.d.). Additionally, designers can augment auditory (temporal) by adding visual labels that lag between realtime.

Slow Temporal Processing Requires Support with Longer Access to Sensory Signal

Again, applying the Channel transformation mechanism to dynamic information could result in the appearance of the information being static by persisting on the screen. This means that the information is frozen or delayed allowing for the additional time to process. An example of this is taking spoken language and presenting it as text on a screen that persists beyond the real time presentation of the words. An example of persistent presentation in vrSocial (Boyd et al., 2018), was to have a visual status bar collecting the time each conversational partner spoke and displaying the updates while maintaining the recent history. Transformed signals for the duration of the conversation could be designed in several other ways as well.

Conclusion

Neuro-inclusive design is designing for variation in human processing systems when designing technology. A key area that impacts many neurodivergent people are differences with dynamically processing multisensory sensory information that build up over time. This includes but is not limited to sensory visual attention, and cognitive processing. These skills that progress from sensory perception to cognitive processing within milliseconds are far more complex than is presented here, however core features are covered. The aim of this Chapter is to make clear the separate but dependent roles to temporal processing and multisensory integration as they relate to sensory processing difficulties in many neurodivergencies. Several strategies are discussed for how to support users through design mechanisms to manage real time interactions so that they can participate, engage and learn. It is my hope that insight into the sensory processing and temporal multisensory integration that designers find inspiration to support neuro inclusive technologies.

References

Ali, S. A., Fadzil, N. A., Reza, F., Mustafar, F., & Begum, T. (2021). A mini review: Visual and auditory perception in dyslexia. *IIUM Medical Journal Malaysia, 20*(4), Article 4. https://doi. org/10.31436/imjm.v20i4.1616

Bionic Reading. (n.d.). https://bionic-reading.com/

Bogdashina, O. (2016). *Sensory perceptual issues in autism and asperger syndrome* (2nd ed.). Jessica Kingsley Publishers.

Boyd, L. E., Gupta, S., Vikmani, S. B., Gutierrez, C. M., Yang, J., Linstead, E., & Hayes, G. R. (2018). vrSocial: Toward Immersive Therapeutic VR Systems for Children with Autism. In *Proceedings of the 2018 CHI Conference on Human Factors in Computing Systems* (pp. 1–12). https:// doi.org/10.1145/3173574.3173778

Brimo, K., Dinkler, L., Gillberg, C., Lichtenstein, P., Lundström, S., & Åsberg Johnels, J. (2021). The co-occurrence of neurodevelopmental problems in dyslexia. *Dyslexia, 27*(3), 277–293. https://doi.org/10.1002/dys.1681

CDC. (2022, June 8). *Data and Statistics About ADHD | CDC.* Centers for Disease Control and Prevention. https://www.cdc.gov/ncbddd/adhd/data.html

CDC. (2023, January 11). *Data and Statistics on Autism Spectrum Disorder | CDC.* Centers for Disease Control and Prevention. https://www.cdc.gov/ncbddd/autism/data.html

Conway, C. M., & Christiansen, M. H. (2005). Modality-constrained statistical learning of tactile, visual, and auditory sequences. *Journal of Experimental Psychology: Learning, Memory, and Cognition, 31*, 24–39. https://doi.org/10.1037/0278-7393.31.1.24

Daft, R. L., & Lengel, R. H. (1986). Organizational information requirements, media richness and structural design. *Management Science, 32*(5), 554–571.

Formoso, M. A., Ortiz, A., Martínez-Murcia, F. J., Brítez, D. A., Escobar, J. J., & Luque, J. L. (2022). Temporal Phase Synchrony Disruption in Dyslexia: Anomaly Patterns in Auditory Processing. In J. M. Ferrández Vicente, J. R. Álvarez-Sánchez, F. de la Paz López, & H. Adeli (Eds.), *Artificial Intelligence in Neuroscience: Affective Analysis and Health Applications* (Vol. 13258, pp. 13–22). Springer International Publishing. https://doi.org/10.1007/978-3-031-06242-1_2

Foss-Feig, J. H., Kwakye, L. D., Cascio, C. J., Burnette, C. P., Kadivar, H., Stone, W. L., & Wallace, M. T. (2010). An extended multisensory temporal binding window in autism spectrum disorders. *Experimental Brain Research, 203*(2), 381–389. https://doi.org/10.1007/s00221-010-2240-4

Franceschini, S., Bertoni, S., Gianesini, T., Gori, S., & Facoetti, A. (2017). A different vision of dyslexia: Local precedence on global perception. *Scientific Reports, 7*(1), Article 1. https://doi. org/10.1038/s41598-017-17626-1

Goldstein-Marcusohn, Y., Goldfarb, L., & Shany, M. (2020). Global and Local Visual Processing in Rate/Accuracy Subtypes of Dyslexia. *Frontiers in Psychology, 11.* https://www.frontiersin.org/ article/https://doi.org/10.3389/fpsyg.2020.00828

Horvitz, E. (1999). Principles of mixed-initiative user interfaces. In *Proceedings of the SIGCHI Conference on Human Factors in Computing Systems* (pp. 159–166). https://doi.org/10.1145/302979. 303030

Hours, C., Recasens, C., & Baleyte, J.-M. (2022). ASD and ADHD comorbidity: What are we talking about? *Frontiers in Psychiatry, 13*, 837424. https://doi.org/10.3389/fpsyt.2022.837424

Humphreys, L. (2005). Cellphones in public: Social interactions in a wireless era. *New Media & Society, 7*(6), 810–833. https://doi.org/10.1177/1461444805058164

Kubovy, M. (1988). Should we resist the seductiveness of the space:Time::Vision:Audition analogy? *Journal of Experimental Psychology: Human Perception and Performance, 14*, 318–320. https://doi.org/10.1037/0096-1523.14.2.318

Kuhl, P. K., & Meltzoff, A. N. (1982). The bimodal perception of speech in infancy. *Science, 218*(4577), 1138–1141. https://doi.org/10.1126/science.7146899

Little, L. M., Dean, E., Tomchek, S., & Dunn, W. (2017). Sensory Processing Patterns in Autism, Attention Deficit Hyperactivity Disorder, and Typical Development. *Physical & Occupational Therapy In Pediatrics, 0*(0), 1–12. https://doi.org/10.1080/01942638.2017.1390809

McCracken, H. S., Murphy, B. A., Glazebrook, C. M., Burkitt, J. J., Karellas, A. M., & Yielder, P. C. (2019). Audiovisual Multisensory Integration and Evoked Potentials in Young Adults With and Without Attention-Deficit/Hyperactivity Disorder. *Frontiers in Human Neuroscience, 13*. https://www.frontiersin.org/articles/https://doi.org/10.3389/fnhum.2019.00095

McGrath, L. M., & Stoodley, C. J. (2019). Are there shared neural correlates between dyslexia and ADHD? A meta-analysis of voxel-based morphometry studies. *Journal of Neurodevelopmental Disorders, 11*(1), 31. https://doi.org/10.1186/s11689-019-9287-8

Meilleur, A., Foster, N. E. V., Coll, S.-M., Brambati, S. M., & Hyde, K. L. (2020). Unisensory and multisensory temporal processing in autism and dyslexia: A systematic review and meta-analysis. *Neuroscience & Biobehavioral Reviews, 116*, 44–63. https://doi.org/10.1016/j.neubiorev.2020.06.013

Mottron, L., Dawson, M., Soulières, I., Hubert, B., & Burack, J. (2006). Enhanced perceptual functioning in autism: an update, and eight principles of autistic perception. *Journal of Autism and Developmental Disorders, 36*(1), 27–43. https://doi.org/10.1007/s10803-005-0040-7

Neurodiversity—NCI (nciglobal, ncienterprise). (2022, April 25). [CgvBlogPost]. https://dceg.cancer.gov/about/diversity-inclusion/inclusivity-minute/2022/neurodiversity

Noel, J.-P., De Niear, M. A., Lazzara, N. S., & Wallace, M. T. (2018). Uncoupling between multisensory temporal function and nonverbal turn-taking in autism spectrum disorder. *IEEE Transactions on Cognitive and Developmental Systems, 10*(4), 973–982. https://doi.org/10.1109/TCDS.2017.2778141

Peterson, R. L., & Pennington, B. F. (2012). Developmental dyslexia. *The Lancet, 379*(9830), 1997–2007. https://doi.org/10.1016/S0140-6736(12)60198-6

Rello, L., & Bigham, J. P. (2017). Good Background Colors for Readers: A Study of People with and Without Dyslexia. In *Proceedings of the 19th International ACM SIGACCESS Conference on Computers and Accessibility* (pp. 72–80). https://doi.org/10.1145/3132525.3132546

Rello, L., & Baeza-Yates, R. (2016). The effect of font type on screen readability by people with dyslexia. *ACM Transactions on Accessible Computing, 8*(4), 1–33. https://doi.org/10.1145/2897736

Robertson, C. E., & Baron-Cohen, S. (2017). Sensory perception in autism. *Nature Reviews Neuroscience, 18*(11), 671–684. https://doi.org/10.1038/nrn.2017.112

Schulze, M., Lux, S., & Philipsen, A. (2020). *Sensory Processing in Adult ADHD – A Systematic Review* [Preprint]. In Review. https://doi.org/10.21203/rs.3.rs-71514/v1

Shinn, J. B. (2003). Temporal processing: The basics. *The Hearing Journal, 56*(7), 52. https://doi.org/10.1097/01.HJ.0000292557.52409.67

Shankweiler, D., & Liberman, I. Y. (1989). Phonology and reading disability: Solving the reading puzzle (Vol. 6). University of Michigan Press

Sonuga-Barke, E., Bitsakou, P., & Thompson, M. (2010). Beyond the dual pathway model: evidence for the dissociation of timing, inhibitory, and delay-related impairments in attention-deficit/hyperactivity disorder. *Journal of the American Academy of Child & Adolescent Psychiatry, 49*(4), 345–355. https://doi.org/10.1016/j.jaac.2009.12.018

Stein, J. (2014). Dyslexia: The role of vision and visual attention. *Current Developmental Disorders Reports, 1*(4), 267–280. https://doi.org/10.1007/s40474-014-0030-6

Stevenson, R. A., Baum, S. H., Segers, M., Ferber, S., Barense, M. D., & Wallace, M. T. (2017). Multisensory speech perception in autism spectrum disorder: From phoneme to whole-word perception. *Autism Research, 10*(7), 1280–1290. https://doi.org/10.1002/aur.1776

Stevenson, R. A., Siemann, J. K., Schneider, B. C., Eberly, H. E., Woynaroski, T. G., Camarata, S. M., & Wallace, M. T. (2014). Multisensory Temporal Integration in Autism Spectrum Disorders. *Journal of Neuroscience, 34*(3), 691–697. https://doi.org/10.1523/JNEUROSCI.3615-13.2014

Wolf, M., & Bowers, P. G. (1999). The double-deficit hypothesis for the developmental dyslexias. *Journal of educational psychology, 91*(3), 415

Neuro-Inclusive Design Considerations for Assistive and Accessible Technologies and Beyond

8

Introduction

The sensory accommodation framework for technology includes descriptions of layers of human sensing and processing involved in learning presented in a hierarchical fashion as is the understanding from a clinical perspective or an educator's perspective. Understanding learning as a collection of skills that are interrelated and interdependent in and of itself could provide some scaffolding for how to develop technologies that have a broad impact, see the learning skills pyramid in Fig. 8.1. As each of these skills is the developmental milestone that is expected in typical development, several of them are also implicated in autism therapies. When someone receives therapy from a system like the school system or an insurance company, often these services are coordinated so that there's a unified plan of service so that each project fits together to support the student or patient with their development where they are currently.

As a previous clinician for over 20 years and now a technologist for a decade, I have observed that this sense of the whole system development is often missed when technologists address only individual skills and focus on single skills as a place of intervention. When someone is not working within a larger team, it is a risky endeavor as inferring the range of dependent skills may not be in place for technologists who are coming into the field of autism from a completely different field and would not know to ask about the underpinnings of all the skills involved. The first chapter is an attempt to highlight the framework that's used in clinical and educational settings and then take it one step further to point out how this aligns with and also contradicts with user-centered design from the perspective of an autistic user who may or may not be interested in the learning pyramid per se. Several examples are given that show a clinical perspective can at times misalign with a user's perspective. The aim of this framework is paired with some careful thought and future discussions that clinicians, caregivers, technologists, autistic users can come

L. Boyd, *The Sensory Accommodation Framework for Technology*, Synthesis Lectures on Technology and Health, https://doi.org/10.1007/978-3-031-48843-6_8

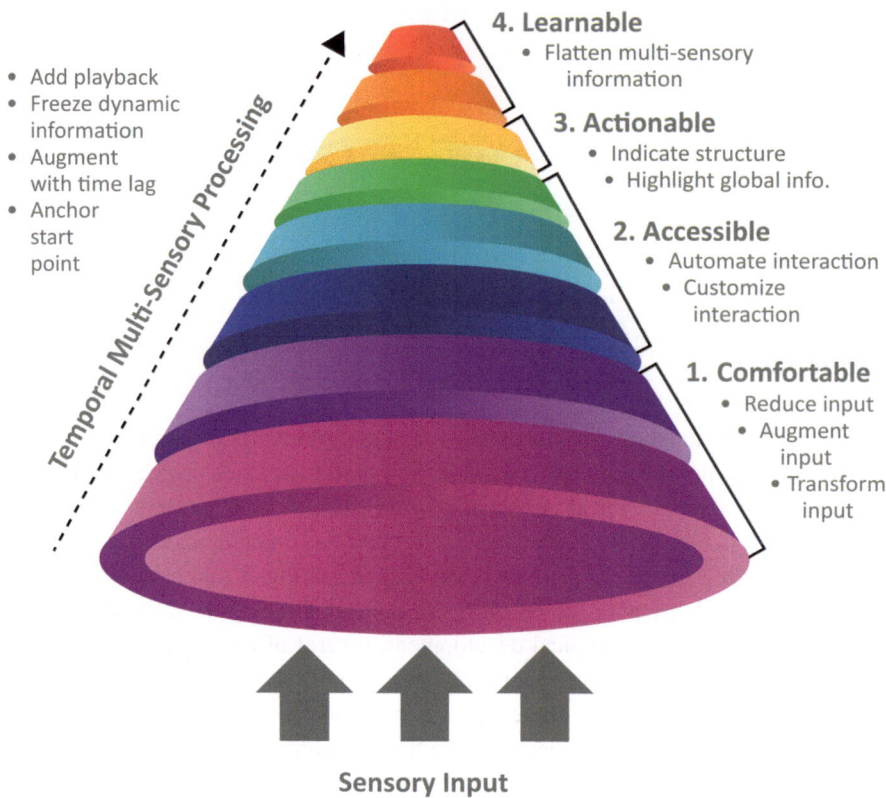

Fig. 8.1 Design guidelines for the sensory accommodation framework

together to design systems that satisfy and hopefully even exceed everyone's expectations. It is quite possible for multiple stakeholders to share a unified vision.

Implications for Designing Neuro-Inclusive Technologies

The interaction design of technologies is a key aspect to the success of a system, systems that are too difficult to use are abandoned and systems that do not support the users desired experiences or abandoned (Dawe, 2006; Deibel, 2013; Shinohara et al., 2018). Therefore, ensuring that the user experience goal is the primary design focus will increase the likelihood that the technology will get adopted. With four main user experience goals for sensory- accommodating technologies, design mechanisms have been described through-out this book and then summarized here, see Fig. 8.1, to inspire user-centered assistive technology for autistic people.

User Experience Goal: Comfortable

The second chapter of this book continues to bridge a clinical view with the user perspective on what a technology might support. After reviewing separate orientations through the two concepts of outward goals (educational or therapeutic technology) from inward goals (assistive and accessible technology). When common goals cannot be reached, the ultimate goal should be that alignment is possible and that user experience goals drive the process. the illustration of user experience goals in Fig. 8.1 top row emphasizes how dependent skills and supports need to be in place in any technology because the person support system is no longer the agent of change and invisible supports that they may have provided are no longer present therefore dependent skills should be assessed and understood to know how a system can provide appropriate accommodations. With this focus that we start at the bottom of the pyramid and work our way up we take a bottom up approach rather than starting at a skill at the top of the pyramid without ensuring that the foundation is solid where we can see how the user goals align with starting at the bottom and assume our first job so as to ensure a technology that is comfortable for use. and then of course going up from there (and in the spirit of Universal Design) making sure that information is perceivable therefore accessible, then actionable and then actually learnable. It is my hope that this becomes a standard in the field for any sensory related technology as at times the developer may not have any lived experience with a sensory difference and therefore not considered in their design. This framework allows for people to think through two sides of the experience with autism—the societal and the personal.

The next goal of this book is taking a deep dive into the sensory processes and the experiences of these differently in autism in Chap. 3. Sensory processing differences have been added to the criteria as part of this lived experience, places for assistive technologists to quickly and systematically glean what these processes are with concrete directions on what to do about it seemed imperative. Often in conference papers there's just as in space to describe the complexity of the human brain and the individual experience that someone has navigating their environment. In this chapter several systems are described and how they may or may not present in someone with autism or any other neurodivergent experience. The aim of this information is to make designers aware of the variety of challenges that exist and the variety of opportunities that exist for designing to support a positive user experience.

Design Considerations for Comfortable Technologies

Consider the perspective of the neurodivergent user in the environment of use, not only their physical environment but the technical and social environment. Ways that the technical environment can support comfort in these spaces is to allow for the reduction of removal of sensory stimuli from the environment. Alternatively, some information may be desired and therefore augmenting the digital environment so that missed information can be recouped would also be appropriate. Lastly, changing the modality of information from a less preferred or sweet channel to a preferred or stronger Channel can make sensory processing more comfortable.

User Experience Goal: Accessible

Chapter four applied background information that's provided in the first three by providing examples of multi-user systems with people that have varied sensory profiles. By showing a range of profiles with different multisensory processing needs, the goal is to show the potential for any system that's used by multiple people to accommodate every need based on individual requirements rather than on any diagnostic label or other labeling mechanism. The VR sensory system that's used as the example in this chapter utilizes a set of sensory accommodations that address not only differences with neurological thresholds to stimulate but also self-regulation behaviors. These are separate processes and are presented as different layers in the sensory accommodation framework. Please see the sensory environment first layer as well as the sensory interaction layer. It is my hope that these could be expanded to include far more mechanisms as well as neurodivergence. These suggestions are just a place to start as I reflect on the last 10 years of my work in this field and speculate about what the next 10 years could bring.

Design Considerations for Accessible Technologies

At the second level from the bottom of the learning cone of the sensory accommodation framework, mechanisms for *adapting the user interaction with the system range from automation to high levels of user control*. These options should be available for everyone but are particularly useful for those who fall on the extreme ends of the self-regulation behavior continuum as indicated in the Sensory Profile 2™ (Dunn, 2014).

User Experience Goal: Actionable

The 5th chapter provided the most specific set of recommendations as it gets down to a sub system of visual processing, specifically visual attention and the hierarchy that's hidden within visual attention known as Global and local processing. This phenomenon has been my area of research for the last five years as I find it fascinating that our brains have separate yet coordinated pathways that break down and regroup information much the way computers do but with intelligence still to be replicated. The global filter is provided as a mechanism for this layer of processing hence at the transition between sensory and cognitive processing and provides a place to consider how to make information actionable. Global and local processing is part of visual attention and visual attention crosses from sensory processing toward cognitive processing. By focusing it at this level in the framework, the rings that are dedicated to some dependents for learning, the aim is still on accessibility so that rapid judgments and attention resources can be allocated without the expectation that something needs to be learned. It's still an automatic process. Expectation that something that happens automatically could be taught may not be reasonable to expect of people while they're also managing the vast and rapid processing that occurs each second. If nothing else, hopefully this framework illustrates at a very abstract level of some of the complexity that occurs in our brains and some of the diversity that exists across the human experience. Visual attention is only one form of attention yet it consumes much of our processing and even has implications for non-visual users who still need to navigate Global and local aspects of stimuli. Much of the current work being done in non-visual technology is starting to address the Gestalt, the whole picture, the metadata, the structure of information and all of these are part of what is available in the physical world from a visual perspective. Having this information organized makes the use of it possible, actionable. Once information is coded as relevant in one's environment, taking action becomes automatic. Higher level skills may not need to be re-learned, rather the accommodation has allowed the user's own abilities to be used. Much of the way information can be transformed to make global and local information obvious in this work has to do with low-level features like spatial frequency and luminance; however, the concept of structuring information by these dimensions applies to non-visual users as well. Previous work highlights how semantic and lexical information can be split for the purpose of making their function clear and disambiguated for non-visual users who may otherwise have to navigate both streams through a single channel of input such as audio from a screen reader (Baldwin et al., 2017).

In the same vein of supporting user experience goals that make information actionable, Chap. 6 is dedicated to the social perception of faces and eyes as experienced by an autistic person. As these are associated with preconscious fear responses and are typically avoided due to potential pain, that information in its current form is not actionable. However, filtering it so that the sensory discomfort is removed and is relieved, the goal of face-to-face interaction for connection can occur, the actions are intact and the barrier to

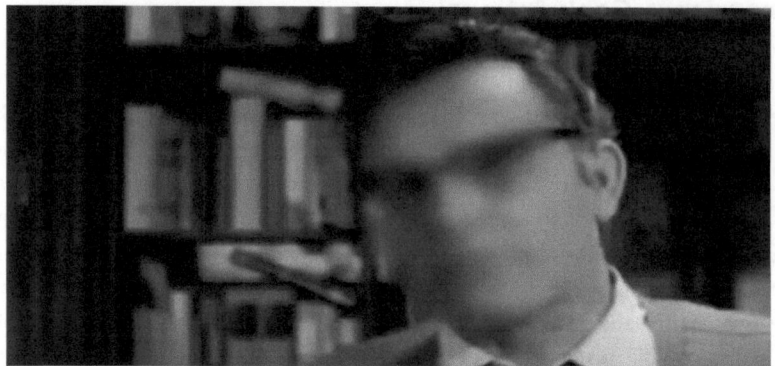

Fig. 8.2 Screenshot of face filter in video as an example of the face blur filter

executing these actions has been addressed. Future work could include ways to transform facial information in a way that is not fear producing. An example here below is a simple filter to blur a face during a movie. My future work will look at users' comfort as well as eye gaze when they view videos with emotional social content that have a mediating filter built in, see Fig. 8.2.

Design Considerations for Actionable Technologies: Make Lean.

To increase the likelihood that user interactions are actionable in a system, a designer can indicate explicitly the structure of information such as global or local. When these two streams of information consist of the same channel, the channel can't be split into two channels for delivering each one with clarity. Alternatively, the levels of information can be reduced to the level that is most appropriate for the task as both global and local processing styles lend themselves to specific tasks.

User Experience Goal: Learnable

These social filters are shown under the learnable level in the sensory accommodation framework and that is because of the level of cognitive processing that goes into a social interaction. By filtering overwhelming sensory information out, the space is provided to form a thought, engage with and learn from the environment.

Design Considerations for Learnable Technologies

The primary suggestion for making information learnable via technology is to flatten multi-sensory information that is difficult to integrate in real time. For example, the flattening multisensory information of the face of a person who is actively talking and moving and expressing through their face by using a blur of the face decreases the burden of integrating multiple messages in real time. It further reduces the need to conserve or switch channels that provide processing power that can be applied to being present in the moment. Another mechanism that supports learnable the user experience goal of learnability is to provide a playback such as an instant replay used televised in professional sports. Customizing the playback speed and duration of viewing could also free up resources to participate in an activity. Lastly, screening out background stimuli (low detection threshold) could support attention on the desired stimulus.

Implication for Temporal MultiSensory Integration Design

The key mechanism for Supporting temporal multisensory integration is temporal transformation (making persistent) of sensory input. Regarding users with a high neurological threshold, flattening and freezing Dynamic information provides time for the information to be processed rather than confusion as the person gets further and further behind in the interaction. A second strategy is to augment the auditory as it is ephemeral. The primary suggestion is to add visual labels and have them lag behind real time so again the person has time to take in the information that this can be done by bolding the first letter of text or adding text to audio. The idea is to create a longer window for the information to be bound thus providing access to the information.

Beyond Sensory Accommodations

Accommodating sensory needs for individual users may address many environmental barriers experienced by neurodivergent users. Addressing barriers beyond an individual user requires attention to social norms that reinforce prejudice and stigma of autistic characteristics. Technologists can address these issues as well and have done so through critical design. However, the audience for critical design is primarily other researchers, where the impact of such work requires additional scaffolding to reach the end user. For this reason, I examine the varying audiences of technologies and propose a new paradigm to intervene on public stigma.

Autism Technologies Ecosystem

Here I describe the autism technology ecosystem, each paradigm has a goal for a specific audience with specific mechanisms for change. Additionally, each paradigm interacts and evolves with the other types over time. I refer to these paradigms as *Assistive, Accessible, Inclusive,* and *Critical*. A new paradigm that I introduce here provides a shift that goes

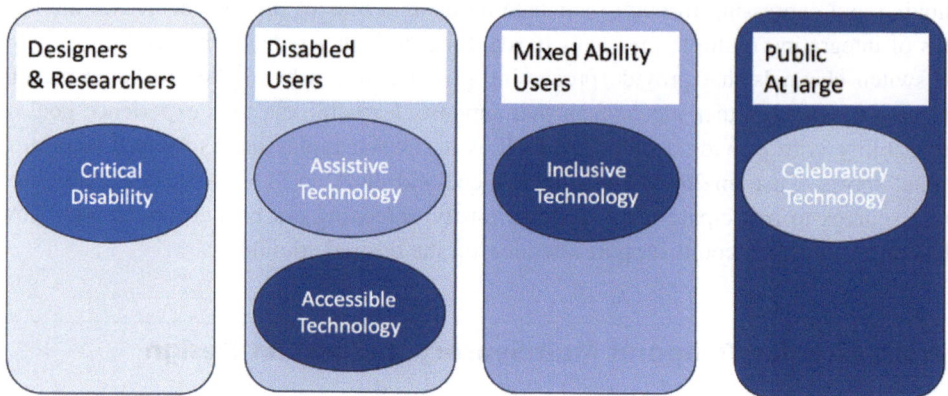

Fig. 8.3 Use cases of autism technology paradigms

beyond interventions that target deficits within the disabled body; environmental barriers for the disabled user; specific accommodations for a collaborative context. Celebratory Technology takes action to address the criticism of existing work. This approach celebrates positive aspects of neurodiversity. Here I add a next evolutionary step by adding Celebratory Technology, see Fig. 8.3.

Any technology in the ecosystem can also be aimed at the public to change perceptions of stigmas, as stigma is a primary barrier to quality of life for autistic people. The goals of each autism technology need not be in competition given that all types of technology are intended to improve the quality of life. Each paradigm targets different audiences and uses different mechanisms. The current paradigms each target personal change whereas Celebratory Technology targets societal change regarding accepting the diversity of human expression. My vision for this new paradigm comes from my professional growth over the past 10 years. I started my career as an autism clinician. After 23 years in that role, I pursued a PhD in Information and Computer Science to extend my impact through innovative interactive technology. As I have published work in each existing paradigm, with recently submitted work in Celebratory Technology described below, I am uniquely qualified to bring to life the next paradigm. Distinctions between the paradigms are described.

Assistive Technology for Autism

The first paradigm is Assistive technology for autism. It has existed for 25 years with the aim to improve deficits that occur *within the person*. The most common of these target social skills from a normative perspective. These technologies are typically based on a medical model of autism which focuses on ways to improve or modulate the ailment within the person. Assistive technologies are for (and sometimes with) disabled users to support a specific need of the user in their daily life. Historically, the skills targeted for improvement through assistive technology were those deemed to be below normative functioning levels. Across a variety of platforms, early interactive technologies targeted communication, social-emotional, academic, life skills, vocational, sensory motor, and restricted and repetitive behavior (Kientz et al., 2013). For example, when targeting reading skills, a clinician or educator might want to change the pronunciation of words in a particular student. Theoretically, the mechanism for change in these types of technologies is often based on learning theory for skill acquisition. My goal when I entered my doctoral program was to apply my deep medical knowledge of autism to develop innovative assistive technologies. I learned that end users may not initiate use of my systems. Instead, it was found that clinicians often drove adoption and use.

Accessible Technology for Autism

Accessible technologies shift the change from within the body or mind to changes in the environment for the purpose of accommodating an impairment. This approach is different from assistive technologies but shares the goal of increasing independence. For example, an accessible technology for reading might provide feedback on a word-by-word basis or develop technology that will give feedback about pronunciation. An example of functionality in accessibility technology is the automating the color of a background to make reading more visible and therefore easier for the user (Rello & Baeza-Yates, 2016; Rello & Bigham, 2017). The burden is on the technology to change the environment and make things easier. Ultimately, the outcome is the same, with the users' reading improving, and with the environmental accommodation version, the user is also likely to be more comfortable. However, this does not replace the benefits of learning to read and proper pronunciation. It is simply a different goal. Theoretically, the mechanism for change in these types of technologies is based on removing barriers to accessing the environment.

Inclusive Technology for Autism

Along with assistive technologies, collaborative and inclusive practices emerged. Inclusive technologies in relation to neurodiversity target collaboration between members in mixed-ability groups, here the examples are of neurodiverse groups. Theoretically, the mechanism for change in these inclusive technologies is the provision of reciprocal support for mixed ability group work, play, or collaboration. Interdependencies between people with varying roles and abilities who work alongside technologies has been brought to the forefront of this space as interdependency adds nuance to inclusive technologies (Bennett et al., 2018). A trailblazer in this domain is *MOSOCO* (Escobedo et al., 2012), a mobile phone app for finding friends at recess connected to elementary students at recess by having everyone use the same mobile application. Additionally, *Incloodle* (Sobel et al., 2016), a collaborative photo-taking app for children of mixed abilities, and my work, *vrSensory* (Boyd, 2019; Boyd et al., 2019), a suite of customized VR environments were built for children with varying types of sensory sensitivities to engage to play environments together. Inclusive technologies aim to support a specific goal of the mixed ability users.

Critical Design for Autism

In contrast to assistive, accessible, and inclusive technologies that target neurodiverse users, critical design targets the scholarship of researchers through analysis of previous works through historical and political injustices. Critical design provides insight that can be the opposite of interventionist products for the purpose of bringing attention to the misalignment between the lived experience and the societal perception of autism.

From a critical disability studies' perspective, assistive technologies perpetuate harmful normalizing behaviors. Critical design brings attention to the misalignment between the lived experience and the societal perception of autism. To draw the designer's attention, critical designs provide critique of the status quo. For example, a parody of interventionist work that was designed to provoke change, called *Facesavr*, describes a face covering that helps allistic (nonautistic) adults be more independent in their emotional processing so the face covering helps one not look at others (Ferdous et al., 2017). From a critical disability studies' perspective, assistive technologies perpetuate harmful normalizing behaviors. Although important, these critical approaches do not necessarily reach the end user in terms of taking direct action to positively impact end users. One publication that is critical yet also contains a pragmatic perspective regarding *Counterventions* (Williams et al., 2023) provides guidelines by reflecting on my previously published assistive technology works to show the evolution from clinicians in assistive technologies to neurodiverse users as the primary stakeholders. The counterventions concept, named from counter-interventions, aims to reduce the likelihood of perpetuating ableism, promoting a "normal" way as the desired way, in interventionist's work by reflectively analyzing through a societal lens. This paradigm addresses the lived experience of disabled people as well as the impact of policy and structural barriers (Williams & Boyd, 2019; Williams et al., 2023). The awareness placed on designers from critical designs projects contributed to this expanded ecosystem and ultimately prompted me to create the new paradigm of Celebratory Technology.

Celebratory Technology for Neurodiversity

Celebratory Technology for Neurodiversity is intended to reduce social stigma by targeting the public at large. Celebratory Technologies aim to support the concept of neurodiversity through the promotion of a positive and broader story of individuals, rather than casting a single, stereotyped story of disability as being "lesser than" with exceptional or ordinary cases of inspiration. The focus here is on appreciating neurodiversity—the reality of the world we all live in—rather than singling out neurodivergence as an exception. Celebratory Technology offers a new paradigm by shifting the burden of change from the neurodivergent person's skillset or providing accommodation for them to changing society's biases at large. Shifting the focus of research outside of the autistic body (and the others involved in their immediate context) creates a new space for design that extends beyond the bodies of a few and calls on all to embrace humanity as a whole.

Conclusion to Book

For a variety of reasons, autistic scholars have said the clinical view of autism needs to be dismantled (Guberman & Haimson, 2023). This book aims to assist with dismantling medical labels and address individual differences across the spectrum of neurodivergence. The Sensory Accommodation framework was devised for autism but has applications for any sensory processing differences. This book is intended to bridge the clinical world to the user experience of autism in a way that provides anyone interested in making therapeutic, educational, assistive, or accessible technologies have a point of entry that is acceptable and needed by all. Future work could extend this Paradigm to add additional mechanisms as a community implements the suggestions within. Additionally, more neurodivergent experiences could be added to the model to expand its impact. As approximately 20% of the world's population may qualify as neurodivergent, these strategies are important for technology designers, users and stakeholders of all types to be aware of and in support of to make the world a more inclusive place.

References

Baldwin, M. S., Hayes, G. R., Haimson, O. L., Mankoff, J., & Hudson, S. E. (2017). The Tangible Desktop: A Multimodal Approach to Nonvisual Computing. *ACM Transactions on Accessible Computing, 10*(3), 9:1–9:28. https://doi.org/10.1145/3075222

Bennett, C. L., Brady, E., & Branham, S. M. (2018). Interdependence as a Frame for Assistive Technology Research and Design. *Proceedings of the 20th International ACM SIGACCESS Conference on Computers and Accessibility*, 161–173. https://doi.org/10.1145/3234695.3236348

124   8 Neuro-Inclusive Design Considerations for Assistive and Accessible ...

Boyd, L., Kendra Day, Kaitlyn Abdo, Ben Wasserman, Gillian Hayes, & Erik Linstead. (2019, May). Paper prototyping comfortable VR play for diverse sensory needs. In *Proceedings of ACM CHI Conference on Human Factors in Computing Systems (CHI'19)*. https://doi.org/10.1145/10.1145/3290607.3313080

Boyd, L. (2019). Designing Sensory-Inclusive Virtual Play Spaces for Children. In *Proceedings of the 18th ACM International Conference on Interaction Design and Children* (pp. 446–451). https://doi.org/10.1145/3311927.3325315

Dawe, M. (2006). Desperately seeking simplicity: How young adults with cognitive disabilities and their families adopt assistive technologies. *Proceedings of the SIGCHI Conference on Human Factors in Computing Systems*, 1143–1152. https://doi.org/10.1145/1124772.1124943

Deibel, K. (2013). A convenient heuristic model for understanding assistive technology adoption. In *Proceedings of the 15th International ACM SIGACCESS Conference on Computers and Accessibility* (pp. 1–2). https://doi.org/10.1145/2513383.2513427

Dunn, W. (2014). Sensory Profile™ 2. Pearson.

Escobedo, L., Nguyen, D. H., Boyd, L., Hirano, S., Rangel, A., Garcia-Rosas, D., Tentori, M., & Hayes, G. (2012). MOSOCO: A mobile assistive tool to support children with autism practicing social skills in real-life situations. *Proceedings of the SIGCHI Conference on Human Factors in Computing Systems*, 2589–2598. https://doi.org/10.1145/2207676.2208649

Ferdous, H. S., Vetere, F., Davis, H., Ploderer, B., O'Hara, K., Comber, R., & Farr-Wharton, G. (2017). Celebratory Technology to Orchestrate the Sharing of Devices and Stories during Family Mealtimes. In *Proceedings of the 2017 CHI Conference on Human Factors in Computing Systems* (pp. 6960–6972). https://doi.org/10.1145/3025453.3025492

Guberman, J., & Haimson, O. (2023). Not robots; Cyborgs—furthering anti-ableist research in human-computer interaction. *First Monday*. https://doi.org/10.5210/fm.v28i1.12910

Kientz, J. A., Goodwin, M. S., Hayes, G. R., & Abowd, G. D. (2013). Interactive technologies for autism. *Synthesis Lectures on Assistive, Rehabilitative, and Health-Preserving Technologies, 2*(2), 1–177. https://doi.org/10.2200/S00533ED1V01Y201309ARH004

Rello, L., & Bigham, J. P. (2017). Good Background Colors for Readers: A Study of People with and Without Dyslexia. In *Proceedings of the 19th International ACM SIGACCESS Conference on Computers and Accessibility* (pp. 72–80). https://doi.org/10.1145/3132525.3132546

Rello, L., & Baeza-Yates, R. (2016). The effect of font type on screen readability by people with dyslexia. *ACM Transactions on Accessible Computing, 8*(4), 1–33. https://doi.org/10.1145/2897736

Shinohara, K., Bennett, C. L., Pratt, W., & Wobbrock, J. O. (2018). Tenets for Social Accessibility: Towards Humanizing Disabled People in Design. *ACM Transactions on Accessible Computing, 11*(1), 1–31. https://doi.org/10.1145/3178855

Sobel, K., Rector, K., Evans, S., & Kientz, J. A. (2016). Incloodle: Evaluating an Interactive Application for Young Children with Mixed Abilities. In *Proceedings of the 2016 CHI Conference on Human Factors in Computing Systems* (pp. 165–176). https://doi.org/10.1145/2858036.2858114

Williams, R. M., & Boyd, L. E. (2019). Prefigurative Politics and Passionate Witnessing. In *The 21st International ACM SIGACCESS Conference on Computers and Accessibility* (pp. 262–266). https://doi.org/10.1145/3308561.3355617

Williams, R. M., Boyd, L., & Gilbert, J. E. (2023). Counterventions: A reparative reflection on interventionist HCI. In *Proceedings of the 2023 CHI Conference on Human Factors in Computing Systems* (pp. 1–11). https://doi.org/10.1145/3544548.3581480